Perspectives in Nursing Management and Care for Older Adults

Series Editors

Julie Santy-Tomlinson
School of Health Sciences
University of Manchester
Manchester, United Kingdom

Paolo Falaschi
Sant'Andrea Hospital
Sapienza University of Rome
Rome, Italy

Karen Hertz
University Hospitals of North Midlands
Royal Stoke University Hospital
Stoke-on-Trent, United Kingdom

W0043033

The aim of this book series is to provide a comprehensive guide to nursing management and care for older adults, addressing specific problems in nursing and allied health professions. It provides a unique resource for nurses, enabling them to provide high-quality care for older adults in all care settings. The respective volumes are designed to provide practitioners with highly accessible information on evidence-based management and care for older adults, with a focus on practical guidance and advice.

Though demographic trends in developed countries are sometimes assumed to be limited to said countries, it is clear that similar issues are now affecting rapidly developing countries in Asia and South America. As such, the series will not only benefit nurses working in Europe, North America, Australasia and many developed countries, but also elsewhere. Offering seminal texts for nurses working with older adults in both inpatient and outpatient settings, it will especially support them during the first five years after nurse registration, as they move towards specialist and advanced practice. The series will also be of value to student nurses, employing a highly accessible style suitable for a broader readership.

More information about this series at http://www.springer.com/series/15860

Gisèle Pickering • Sandra Zwakhalen
Sharon Kaasalainen
Editors

Pain Management in Older Adults

A Nursing Perspective

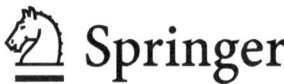 Springer

Editors
Gisèle Pickering
CIC Inserm 1405
University Clermont Auvergne and
University Hospital
Clermont-Ferrand
France

Sandra Zwakhalen
Health Services Research
Maastricht University Health Services
Research
Maastricht
Limburg
The Netherlands

Sharon Kaasalainen
School of Nursing
McMaster University School of Nursing
Hamilton
Ontario
Canada

ISSN 2522-8838   ISSN 2522-8846   (electronic)
Perspectives in Nursing Management and Care for Older Adults
ISBN 978-3-030-10094-0   ISBN 978-3-319-71694-7   (eBook)
https://doi.org/10.1007/978-3-319-71694-7

This Springer imprint is published by Springer Nature, under the registered company Springer International Publishing AG
The registered company address is: Gewerbestrasse 11, 6330 Cham, Switzerland

Preface

The book *Pain Management in Older Adults: A Nursing Perspective* features theoretical and practical information about the assessment and management of pain in older adults. It is written for nurses, nurse specialists, advanced nurse practitioners, and academics who are interested in pain management in older adults.

Pain is one of the most distressing and commonest symptoms of later life. Mood, quality of life, independence, and relationship are all affected and the high prevalence of pain has a substantial impact at both individual and societal level. Although more attention has been paid to pain in older persons over the last decades, pain remains underdetected, underestimated, and undertreated especially in the most vulnerable with neurodegenerative disorders and communication difficulties.

Nurses care for older people in primary, secondary, and independent settings and have been at the forefront of pain care for centuries. Nurses play a crucial role in the assessment and management of pain. Their involvement with older persons is multifaceted, involved in pain assessment, comfort care, nonpharmacological and pharmacological approaches, and beyond managing an individual's pain, critical self-reflection and service development. Nurses are deeply involved throughout the care process and collaborate with interdisciplinary teams throughout care settings. Nursing older people is challenging and rewarding and we felt it was timely to produce a book from the nursing perspective.

We have included chapters covering epidemiology, assessment, therapeutic approaches, as well as chapters focused on the pivotal role of nurses in older persons pain management.

The editors and authors have worked to ensure that these chapters reflect older adults pain management essentials. It is our hope that this book will provide nurses working in primary health and care social areas as well as undergraduate and postgraduate nursing students with evidence that helps them in the caring process.

The book is an international collaborative effort and the editors would like to express their gratitude to all the authors for their contributions.

Clermont-Ferrand, France   Gisèle Pickering
Maastricht, The Netherlands   Sandra Zwakhalen
Hamilton, ON, Canada   Sharon Kaasalainen

Contents

Abbreviations

°C	Degree Celsius
5-HTR	Serotonin receptor
ABCDEF	Awakening and Breathing coordination of daily sedation and ventilator removal trials; Choice of sedative or analgesic exposure; Delirium monitoring and management; Early mobility and exercise and Family-centered care
ACC	Anterior cingulate cortex
ACR	American College of Rheumatology
AD	Alzheimer disease
ADL	Activities of daily living
AEs	Adverse effects
AGS	American Geriatrics Society
AI	Appreciative Inquiry
AMDA	American Medical Directors Association
AMPA	α-amino-3-hydroxy-5-methyl-4-isoxazolepropionic acid
APN	Advanced practice nursing
ASPMN	American Society for Pain Management Nursing
ATP	Adenosine triphosphate
AuPS	Australian Pain Society
B2 receptor	Bradykinin receptor 2
BDNF	Brain-derived neurotrophic factor
BGS	British Geriatrics Society
BPGs	Best practice guidelines
BPS	British Pain Society
BPS scale	Behavioral pain scale
BPS-NI	Behavioral pain scale—not intubated
BPSD	Behavioral and psychological symptoms of dementia
Ca^{2+}	Calcium ion
CAM	Confusion assessment method
CAM-ICU	CAM for intensive care
CaMKII	Calcium-calmodulin kinase II
cAMP	Cyclic adenosine monophosphate
CAMs	Complementary and alternative therapies
CBT	Cognitive behavioral therapy
CCK	Cholecystokinin

CGRP	Calcitonin gene-related peptide
CNPI	Checklist of nonverbal pain indicators
CNS	Central nervous system
Coxibs	Cyclooxygenase-II selective inhibitors
CPAT	Certified nursing assistant pain assessment tool
CPGs	Clinical practice guidelines
CPOT	Critical-care pain observation tool
CPS	Canadian Pain Society
CREB	cAMP response element binding protein
CT scan	Computerized tomography scan
DNA	Desoxyribonucleic acid
DNIC	Diffuse noxious inhibitory controls
DOR	Delta opioid receptor
DQP	Deutsches Netzwerk für Qualitätssicherung in der Pflege
DRG	Dorsal root ganglion
DSM-5	Diagnostic and Statistical Manual of Mental Disorders Fifth Edition
DVT	Deep vein thromboembolism
DZNE	German Center for Neurodegenerative Diseases
eCASH	Early Comfort using Analgesia, minimal Sedatives and maximal Human care
EPSP	Excitatory postsynaptic potential
ERK	Extracellular signal-regulated protein kinase
fMRI	Functional magnetic resonance imaging
GABA	Gamma-aminobutyric acid
GP	General practitioner
H^+	Hydrogen ion
H1	Histamine receptor
HCP	Health care practitioner
IASP	International Association for the Study of Pain
ICU	Intensive care unit
ID	Intellectual disabilities
IPSP	Inhibitory postsynaptic potential
IQ	Intellectual quotient
IV	Intravenous
KA	Kainate
KOR	Kappa opioid receptor
KT	Knowledge translation
LPNs	Licensed practical nurses
MCI	Mild cognitive impairment
mGluR	Metabotropic glutamate receptors
MMSE	Mini-mental state examination
MOBID	Mobilization-observation-behavior-intensity-dementia pain scale
MOR	Mu opioid receptor
Na^+	Sodium ion
NCCIH	National Center for Complementary and Integrative Health

NHS	National Health Service
NICE	National Institute for Health and Care Excellence
NMDA	N-methyl-D-aspartate
NOPPAIN	Non-communicative patient's pain assessment instrument
NPs	Nurse practitioners
NRM	Nucleus raphe magnus
NRS	Numerical rating scale
NSAIDs	Nonsteroidal anti-inflammatory drugs
PACSLAC	Pain assessment checklist for seniors with limited ability to communicate
PAG	Periaqueductal grey
PAINAD	Pain assessment in advanced dementia
PARIHS	Promoting Action on Research Implementation in Health Services
PATs	Pain assessment tools
PBOICIE	Pain behaviors for osteoarthritis instrument for cognitively impaired elders
PET	Positron emission tomography
PFC	Prefrontal cortex
PKA	Protein kinase A
PKC	Protein kinase C
PLC	Phospholipase C
PMN	Pain management nursing
QI	Quality Initiatives
RASS	Richmond agitation sedation scale
RCTs	Randomized clinical trials
RNAO	Registered Nurses Association of Ontario
RNs	Registered nurses
RVM	Rostral ventromedial medulla
S1	Primary somatosensory cortex
S2	Secondary somatosensory cortex
SRD	Subnucleus reticularis dorsalis
TENS	Transcutaneous electrical nerve stimulation
TRP	Transient receptor potential cation channel
TRPM8	Transient receptor potential cation channel subfamily M member 8
TRPV	Transient receptor potential vanilloid
TTX	Voltage-gated sodium channel
TTXr	Tetrodotoxin-resistant sodium channels
UK	United Kingdom
UTI	Urinary tract infection
VAS	Visual analogue scale
VDS	Verbal descriptor scale
VIP	Vasoactive intestinal peptide
VRS	Verbal rating scale
WDR	Wide dynamic range
WHO	World Health Organization

Gisèle Pickering

Abstract

In both developed and developing countries, populations are aging, largely due to a significant increase in life expectancy. This phenomenon will continue to progress over the next few decades. Chronic pain is the most frequently reported symptom in community settings, where most older people liven, as well as in residential care units. Pain is accompanied by heterogeneous comorbidities and dramatically impairs the quality of life of older people. Pain management is particularly difficult in older people with communication disorders, and this public health problem remains overall underrecognized and undertreated.

1.1 Prevalence of Pain in the Aging Population

Population aging is taking place worldwide; the increasingly greater life expectancy has been driven, in part, by reduced mortality at older ages. Global projections suggest that the proportion of older people (age 60 years and older) will rise from 12.3% in 2015 to 16.5% in 2030 and 21.5% in 2050 (UNDESA 2015). Consequently, the estimated 46.8 million people worldwide living with dementia in 2015 will almost double every 20 years, reaching 131.5 million in 2050 (https://www.alz.co.uk/research/statistics). Epidemiological and retrospective studies of several somatic and visceral pathological conditions (Breivik et al. 2006; Pickering et al.

G. Pickering
Department of Clinical Pharmacology, University Regional Hospital,
Clermont-Ferrand, France

Inserm CIC 1405 and Neurodol 1107, Medical Faculty, Clermont-Ferrand, Cedex, France
e-mail: gisele.pickering@uca.fr

© Springer International Publishing AG, part of Springer Nature 2018
G. Pickering et al. (eds.), *Pain Management in Older Adults*, Perspectives in Nursing
Management and Care for Older Adults, https://doi.org/10.1007/978-3-319-71694-7_1

2001; de Tommaso et al. 2016) report that the prevalence of pain in older people is very high. An age-related increase in the prevalence of chronic pain, at least until the age of 70, has been reported, although the nature and type of pain may differ from that of younger adults. Pain due to degenerative diseases, osteoarthritis, cancer and neuropathic conditions such as diabetic neuropathy, postherpetic neuralgia and post-stroke are much more common (Pickering and Leplege 2011; Miranda et al. 2012). Despite differences in the absolute prevalence of chronic pain, depending on methodological differences between studies, a peak prevalence has been reported during late middle age (50–65 years, 20–80%) followed by a plateau (65–85 years, 20–70%) and then a decline in very advanced age (85+ years, 25–60%) (Gibson and Lussier 2012; Abdulla et al. 2013). Pain is common in older individuals (American Geriatrics Society [AGS] Panel on Persistent Pain in Older Persons 2002). Several studies have shown that approximately 14% of older adults suffer from moderate to severe, continuous pain, occurring on most days throughout the previous 3 months (Breivik et al. 2006; Smith et al. 2001). Those over 75 years were found to be four times more likely to suffer from significant pain when compared to younger adults.

Causes of pain can be acute or chronic. Acute painful conditions are very frequent, as older people have the highest rates of surgery, procedural pain, and complications (Macintyre and Schug 2007), and chronic conditions disproportionately affect older adults (Pickering et al. 2001; Pickering and Leplege 2011; Pickering and Herpes Zoster and Functional Decline Consortium 2015). Chronic and persistent pain appear to have a very high prevalence; 58–83% of residents in long-term care facilities (Abdulla et al. 2013; Takai et al. 2010) with 3.7% report excruciating pain on at least 1 day in the previous week (Teno et al. 2004). The prevalence of neuropathic pain, a persistent type of chronic pain, has been underestimated in older people for many years (Pickering et al. 2016). It is now estimated to affect 20% of persons with osteoarthritis (French et al. 2017) and up to 48% of community-dwelling older people (Rapo-Pylkkö et al. 2015). Persistent neuropathic pain results in functional decline and loss of autonomy (Pickering and Herpes Zoster and Functional Decline Consortium 2015).

Although pain is very common in older adults, there is also clear evidence of atypical pain presentations, including a relative absence of pain symptoms. For instance, myocardial pain is much less common in older adults, with 35–42% of adults over the age of 65 years experiencing apparently silent or painless myocardial infarction (Hwang et al. 2009). Physiological/biological changes may be involved, but evidence also shows that older people have increased stoicism, are more likely to accept mild aches and pains and have altered pain beliefs and attitudes (Gibson 2005). In older adults suffering from dementia, atypical presentations of pain may also occur due to the type of dementia and associated neuropathological changes. For example, dementia with Lewy bodies may reduce the person's facial expression and may, therefore, affect the facial response to pain. A systematic review determined the prevalence of pain for each of the four major dementia subtypes (Alzheimer's disease, vascular dementia, frontotemporal dementia and dementia with Lewy bodies) in a community setting and long-term care facilities. Study findings demonstrated that the prevalence of pain did not differ significantly between dementia subtypes, although this was probably due to neuropathological changes. An overall high prevalence of pain in dementia was found, without significant differences between the dementia subtypes, varying from 46% for Alzheimer's disease and up to 56% for vascular dementia (van Kooten et al. 2016).

1.2   Pain and Comorbidities

Depression and anxiety can interact with pain and cognitive functioning. Normally, prevalence of depression and anxiety declines with aging except when comorbid with persistent pain (Baker et al. 2017). Estimates of prevalence of depression and anxiety jump significantly in samples with comorbid medical illnesses and anxiety symptoms occurring in 36–85% of pathologies (e.g. cardiac, cancer, pulmonary, diabetes) (Wolitzky-Taylor et al. 2010), most of which are more common in older adults, while 32–54% of patients with chronic pain have a major depressive disorder (Banks and Kerns 1996).

Pain itself can also have major deleterious effects on cognitive performance, and deficits in attention, working memory and mental flexibility are instigated by the presence of pain (Abeare et al. 2010; Weiner et al. 2006; Lee et al. 2010). It is probable that both pain and its related psychosocial problems (depression, sleep disturbance, opioid use) have an influence on deficits in cognition. Cognition itself may be altered with aging, ranging from mild cognitive impairment (MCI) (an impairment in both memory and non-memory cognitive domains) (Roberts and Knopman 2013) to dementias (Small et al. 1997). Pain assessment and care in patients with dementia or patients with communication disorders are particularly difficult (Eccleston 2017), as they have potential changes in the pain experience and have their own unique pain-related impacts on mood, behaviour and drug treatment.

Pain is identified in 43% of verbally communicative residents compared to only 17% of patients verbally non-communicative (Sengstaken and King 1993), offering a potential explanation for why prevalence estimates of pain are reduced in those with dementia (Eritz and Hadjistavropoulos 2011; van Herk et al. 2009). Several studies have confirmed that patients with severe cognitive impairment demonstrate the strongest relationship between pain and depression (Achterberg et al. 2010; Kenefick 2004; Jensen-Dahm et al. 2012).

The occurrence of behavioural and psychological symptoms of dementia (BPSD) has long been noted. Higher levels of agitation or aggression have consistently been shown to be associated with pain (Husebo et al. 2011; Pelletier and Landreville 2007) in these vulnerable people, but the current pool of knowledge in the large area of pain and dementia remains incomplete.

Conclusion

While, today, 18–20% of the elderly live in long-term care settings and nursing homes, a variable percentage are transiently present in hospitals, palliative care units and accident and emergency departments. Most older people live in the community. For affective reasons, as well as from the point of view of state finances, the current policy is to 'age in place'; older adults are encouraged to remain in their own chosen environment for as long as possible. Older people present a very large heterogeneity in physical health, mental status and settings, and recurring barriers to adequate pain management (Savvas and Gibson 2015; Pickering 2016; Eccleston, 2017) now need to be fully identified. Available data, although limited, tell us that nursing staff are not well educated in aspects of geriatric pain. The nurse caring for older adults in pain must understand the special needs of this vulnerable population to be able to provide person-centred, safe and effective care.

References

Abdulla A, Adams N, Bone M, Elliott AM, Gaffin J, Jones D, Knaggs R, Martin D, Sampson L, Schofield P, British Geriatric Society. Guidance on the management of pain in older people. Age Ageing. 2013;42(Suppl 1):i1–57.

Abeare CA, Cohen JL, Axelrod BN, Leisen JC, Mosley-Williams A, Lumley MA. Pain, executive functioning, and affect in patients with rheumatoid arthritis. Clin J Pain. 2010;26(8):683–9.

Achterberg WP, Gambass GI, Finne-Soveri H, Liperoti R, Noro A, et al. Pain in European long-term care facilities: cross-National Study in Finland, Italy and The Netherlands. Pain. 2010;148:70–4.

American Geriatrics Society [AGS] Panel on Persistent Pain in Older Persons. The management of persistent pain in older persons. J Am Geriatr Soc. 2002;50(Suppl 6):S205–24.

Baker KS, Gibson SJ, Georgiou-Karistianis N, Giummarra MJ. Relationship between self-reported cognitive difficulties, objective neuropsychological test performance and psychological distress in chronic pain. Eur J Pain. 2017;21:601–13.

Banks SM, Kerns RD. Explaining high rates of depression in chronic pain: a diathesis-stress framework. Psychol Bull. 1996;119:95–110.

Breivik H, Collett B, Ventafridda V, Cohen R, Gallacher D. Survey of chronic pain in Europe: prevalence, impact on daily life, and treatment. Eur J Pain. 2006;10(4):287–333.

de Tommaso M, Arendt-Nielsen L, Defrin R, Kunz M, Pickering G, Valeriani M. Pain assessment in neurodegenerative diseases. Behav Neurol. 2016;2016:2949358.

Eccleston C, editor. Pickering pain and geriatrics in Europe in European pain management. Oxford: Oxford University Press; 2017.

Eritz H, Hadjistavropoulos T. Do informal caregivers consider nonverbal behavior when they assess pain in people with severe dementia? J Pain. 2011;12:331–9.

French HP, Smart KM, Doyle F. Prevalence of neuropathic pain in knee or hip osteoarthritis: a systematic review and meta-analysis. Semin Arthritis Rheum. 2017;47(1):1–8.

Gibson SJ. Age differences in psychological factors related to pain perception and report. In: Gibson SJ, Wiener DK, editors. Pain in older adults. Seattle: IASP Press; 2005. p. 87–110.

Gibson SJ, Lussier D. Prevalence and relevance of pain in older persons. Pain Med. 2012;13:S23–6.

Husebo BS, Ballard C, Sandvik R, Nilsen OB, Aarsland D. Efficacy of treating pain to reduce behavioural disturbances in residents of nursing homes with dementia: cluster randomised clinical trial. BMJ. 2011;343:d4065.

Hwang SY, Park EH, Shin ES, Jeong MH. Comparison of factors associated with atypical symptoms in younger and older patients with acute coronary syndromes. J Korean Med Sci. 2009;24(5):789–94.

Jensen-Dahm C, Vogel A, Waldorff FB, Waldemar G. Discrepancy between self- and proxy-rated pain in Alzheimer's disease: results from the Danish Alzheimer Intervention Study. J Am Geriatr Soc. 2012;60:1274–8.

Kenefick AL. Pain treatment and quality of life: reducing depression and improving cognitive impairment. J Gerontol Nurs. 2004;30:22–9.

Lee DM, Pendleton N, Tajar A, O'Neill TW, O'Connor DB, Bartfai G, et al. Chronic widespread pain is associated with slower cognitive processing speed in middle-aged and older European men. Pain. 2010;151(1):30–6.

Macintyre PE, Schug SA. Acute pain management: a practical guide. 3rd ed. Saunders Elsevier: Edinburgh; 2007.

Miranda VS, Decarvalho VB, Machado LA, Dias JM. Prevalence of chronic musculoskeletal disorders in elderly Brazilians: a systematic review of the literature. BMC Musculoskelet Disord. 2012;13:82.

Pelletier IC, Landreville P. Discomfort and agitation in older adults with dementia. BMC Geriatr. 2007;7:27.

Pickering G. In: Gibson S, Lautenbacher S, editors. "Pharmacological treatment", chapter in "pain and dementia". Washington, DC: IASP Press; 2016.

Pickering G, Herpes Zoster and Functional Decline Consortium. Functional decline and herpes zoster in older people: an interplay of multiple factors. Aging Clin Exp Res. 2015;27(6): 757–65.

Pickering G, Leplege A. Herpes zoster, postherpetic neuralgia and quality of life. Pain Pract. 2011;11:397–402.

Pickering G, Deteix A, Eschalier A, Dubray C. Impact of pain of nursing home residents on their recreational activities. Aging. 2001;13:44–8.

Pickering G, Marcoux M, Chapiro S, David L, Rat P, Michel M, Bertrand I, Voute M, Wary B. An algorithm for neuropathic pain management in older people. Drugs Aging. 2016;33(8): 575–83.

Rapo-Pylkkö S, et al. Neuropathic pain among community-dwelling older people: a clinical study in Finland. Drugs Aging. 2015;32:737–42.

Roberts R, Knopman DS. Classification and epidemiology of MCI. Clin Geriatr Med. 2013;29(4):753–72.

Savvas S, Gibson S. Pain management in residential aged care facilities. Aust Fam Physician. 2015;44(4):198–203.

Sengstaken EA, King SA. The problems of pain and its detection among geriatric nursing home residents. J Am Geriatr Soc. 1993;41:541–4.

Small GW, Rabins PV, Barry PP, et al. Diagnosis and treatment of Alzheimer disease and related disorders. Consensus statement of the American Association for Geriatric Psychiatry, the Alzheimer's Association, and the American Geriatrics Society. JAMA. 1997;278:1363–71.

Smith BH, Elliott AM, Chambers WA, Smith WC, Hannaford PC, Penny K. The impact of chronic pain in the community. Fam Pract. 2001;18(3):292–9.

Takai Y, Yamamoto-Mitani N, Okamoto Y, Koyama K, Honda A. Literature review of pain prevalence among older residents of nursing homes. Pain Manag Nurs. 2010;11(4):209–23.

Teno JM, Kabumoto G, Wetle T, Roy J, Mor V. Daily pain that was excruciating at some time in the previous week: prevalence, characteristics, and outcomes in nursing home residents. J Am Geriatr Soc. 2004;52(5):762–7.

UNDESA. Population division, World population prospects: the 2015 revision, DVD Edition; 2015.

van Herk R, van Dijk M, Biemold N, Tibboel D, Baar FPM, de Wit R. Assessment of pain: can caregivers or relatives rate pain in nursing home residents? J Clin Nurs. 2009;18:2478–85.

van Kooten J, Binnekade TT, van der Wouden JC, Stek ML, Scherder EJ, Husebø BS, Smalbrugge M, Hertogh CM. A review of pain prevalence in Alzheimer's, vascular, frontotemporal and Lewy body dementias. Dement Geriatr Cogn Disord. 2016;41(3-4):220–32.

Weiner DK, Rudy TE, Morrow L, Slaboda J, Lieber S. The relationship between pain, neuropsychological performance and physical function in community-dwelling older adults with chronic low back pain. Pain Med. 2006;7:60–70.

Wolitzky-Taylor KB, Castriotta N, Lenze EJ, Stanley MA, Craske MG. Anxiety disorders in older adults: a comprehensive review. Depress Anxiety. 2010;27(2):190–211.

Elodie Martin

Abstract

While acute pain is an alarm signal involving unpleasant sensations and vegeta-tive and behavioural reactions, chronic pain presents with long-lasting conse-quences. The underlying mechanisms of pain chronicization after an acute pain episode involve both peripheral and central nervous system sensitization. In this chapter, the pathophysiology of acute and chronic pain will be described with a specific focus on elderly patients. Ageing is accompanied by physiological changes, and acute and chronic pain are a major concern for older people. Knowledge of the clinical manifestations of pain processing changes in older people is essential in guaranteeing optimal pain management.

2.1 Definitions of Pain

Pain is defined internationally as "an unpleasant sensory and emotional experience associated with actual or potential tissue damage, or described in terms of such dam-age" (IASP Task Force on Taxonomy 1994). Another definition was provided by McCaffery and Beebe in 1989: "Pain is whatever the experiencing person says it is, existing whenever the experiencing person say it does" (McCaffery and Beebe 1989). These definitions highlight that pain is a complex subjective experience, involving physiological and neuropsychological domains. However, the definition of McCaffery and Beebe is not applicable to individuals with cognitive impairment or inability to communicate verbally and who are unable to express and report their pain.

E. Martin
Clinical Pharmacology Center, Clinical Research Center Inserm 1405,
University Hospital, Medical Faculty, F-63003 Clermont-Ferrand cedex, France
e-mail: e-martin@chu-clermontferrand.fr

© Springer International Publishing AG, part of Springer Nature 2018
G. Pickering et al. (eds.), *Pain Management in Older Adults*, Perspectives in Nursing
Management and Care for Older Adults, https://doi.org/10.1007/978-3-319-71694-7_2

Pain is distinguished from nociception which is a manifestation of a neurophysiological protection system that aims to detect internal (visceral origin) or external (cutaneous) stimuli of intensity that threatens the physical integrity of the individual. As well as sensory aspects, pain also includes psychological and social aspects (Gatchel et al. 2007). The sensory (or somatic) component of the "pain" signal represents the neurophysiological processes of detection, qualitative definition, topographical location and intensity quantification. The psychological (or emotional) component relates to the affective, unpleasant and sometimes unbearable sensation that accompanies pain. This dimension of the pain experience is the most severe and is responsible for the anxio-depressive symptoms when pain is recurrent or persistent.

Pain may be defined as acute or chronic. In healthcare practice, different types of acute and chronic pain can be encountered depending on their origin and duration (IASP Task Force on Taxonomy 1994; Millan 1999). Acute pain is considered as recently established pain and transient and reversible when the causal lesion is treated and may follow moderate trauma. Acute pain can be considered "useful" as it informs the development of an external or internal lesion (Carr and Goudas 1999). In comparison to acute pain, which resolves when healing is complete, chronic pain is described as a multidimensional syndrome that persists despite the termination of the healing process. It is mainly characterized by its duration, conventionally more than 3 months (a length of time more than 6 months is often preferred for research purposes) (IASP Taxonomy Working Group 2011), but also by the psychological repercussions that impact the mood (anxiety, depression), daily activities (physical, professional, social and family) and quality of life.

Pain is also defined as nociceptive, neuropathic, inflammatory and nociplastic. Nociceptive pain is usually a result of excessive stimulation of skin and internal organ nociceptors (sensory receptors for pain) and occurs with a normally functioning somatosensory system. Inflammatory pain is often of internal origin (e.g. due to infection, osteoarthritis, digestive pain). Neuropathic pain is caused by a lesion or disease of the peripheral or central somatosensory nervous system. Nociplastic (psychogenic or dysfunctional) pain does not have a clearly identifiable somatic origin, but is mainly caused by psychological factors. John Loeser (1982), in his model of pain, proposes four pain dimensions: nociception, pain, suffering and pain behaviour (Fig. 2.1); in addition, physical aspects of the pain experience and biopsychosocial factors play an important role in the understanding of pain and suffering.

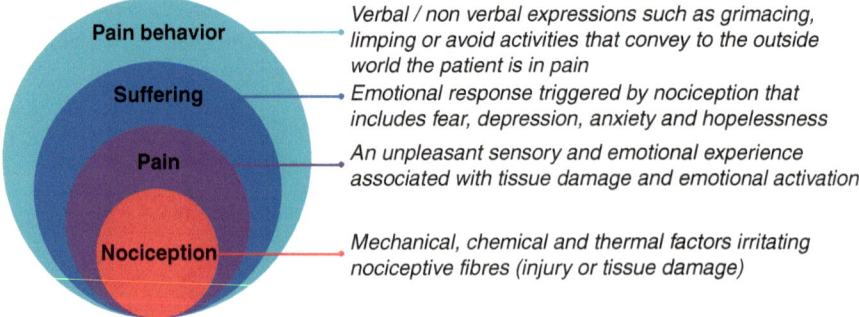

Fig. 2.1 Loeser's model of pain

The nervous system detects and interprets a wide range of thermal and mechanical stimuli, as well as environmental or endogenous irritant chemicals. When they are intense, these stimuli generate acute pain. With chronic pain, the peripheral and central nervous system structures involved in the transmission of pain can undergo plasticity with synaptic reorganization and structural remodelling.

2.2   Acute Pain

Acute nociceptive impulses involve complex electrophysiological and neurochemical mechanisms (Millan 1999), and different steps are described: (1) development of the nociceptive impulse, caused by various stimuli (thermal, mechanical, chemical, electrical), signal transduction at the nociceptor site and signal conduction along the primary afferent nerve fibre; (2) signal relay and modulation at the dorsal horn of the spinal cord towards supraspinal sites; and (3) signal integration at the supraspinal level where the nociceptive impulse is transformed into a conscious message: a painful sensation with a sensory-discriminative component (localization, intensity,

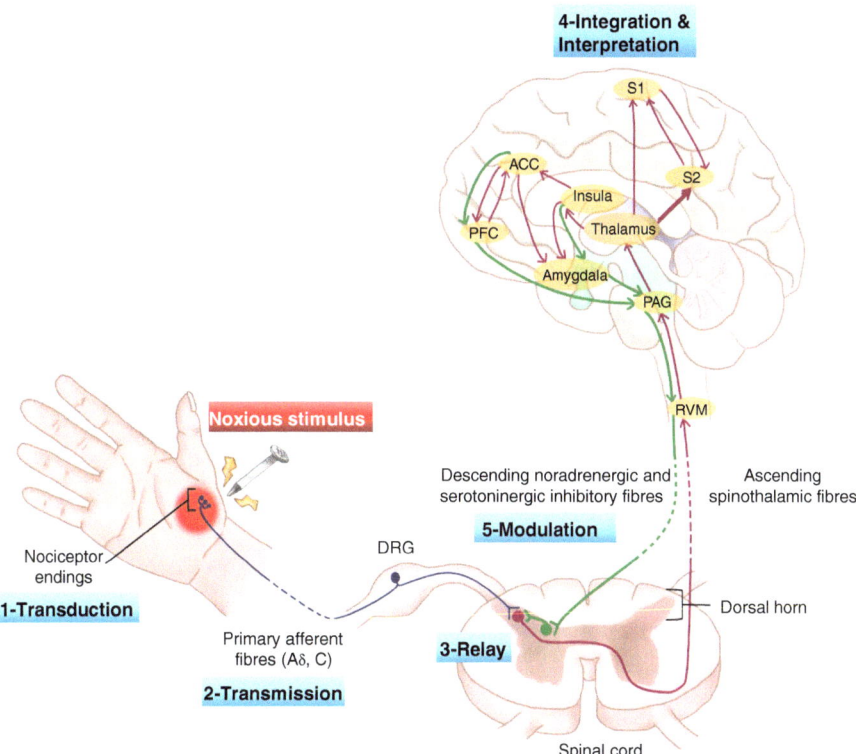

Fig. 2.2 Pain processing and modulation pathways (*ACC* anterior cingulate cortex, *DRG* dorsal root ganglion, *PAG* periaqueductal grey, *PFC* prefrontal cortex, *RVM* rostral-ventromedial medulla, *S1* primary somatosensory cortex, *S2* secondary somatosensory cortex)

duration of the nociceptive stimulus) and an emotional and affective component which transmits the unpleasant characteristics of the pain (Fig. 2.2).

2.2.1 Peripheral Mechanisms

2.2.1.1 Nociceptors and Primary Afferent Fibres

Nociceptors are peripheral sensory receptors found in most tissues (skin, viscera, muscle, cartilage) and which respond to nociceptive stimuli. In skin, nociceptors are small-diameter Aδ-fibres (2–6 μm) that are thinly myelinated and have moderate conduction velocity (12–30 m/s) and small-diameter unmyelinated C-fibres (0.4–1.2 μm) that are free nerve endings with slow conduction velocity (0.5–2 m/s). Aδ- and C-fibres represent respectively 10% and 70% of sensory fibres (Millan 1999).

Following a nociceptive stimulation, two consecutive pain sensations are described. The first, almost immediate and short-lasting, is described as sharp and corresponds to the rapid transmission of epicritic sensitivity conveyed by the Aδ-fibres. The second is transmitted by C-fibres and is perceived, 1–2 s later, as a diffuse and burning painful sensation. Some classes of Aδ and C nociceptors respond to mechanical or thermal stimuli or both. Other receptors respond to chemical stimulation, while some "silent" nociceptors respond only to tissue injury or inflammation (Dubin and Patapoutian 2010). In order to transduct the nociceptive message along the peripheral nerve fibre, the mechanical, thermal and chemical stimuli must be transformed into action potentials. Thus, specific transducers are involved as channel receptors. Among these, transient receptor potential cation channels (TRP channels) are sensitive to temperature. Transient receptor potential vanilloid channels TRPV1 (C-fibres, 43 °C activation threshold) and TRPV2 (Aδ-fibres, 53 °C activation threshold) are sensitive to nociceptive temperature and nociceptive mechanical stimuli (Danigo et al. 2013). TRPV3 (C-fibres, 32 °C activation threshold) and TRPV4 receptors (C-fibres, 24 °C activation threshold) are, instead, responsible for non-warm nociceptive sensations. Non-nociceptive and nociceptive cold sensations can be encoded by the TRPM8 (sensitive to menthol and temperature range of 8–28 °C) and the TTXR Nav1.8 (tetrodotoxin-resistant) channels. TRP may also be sensitive to exogenous and algogenic chemicals such as chili pepper (capsaicin), acidity (H^+ hydrogen ion) and some venoms which can alter the conformation of receptors and lower their activation threshold (Dubin and Patapoutian 2010).

2.2.1.2 Algogenic Substances Responsible for Nociceptor Sensitization

Following tissue injury, many sensitizing algogenic substances are released and are followed by the inflammatory process which is initiated by mast cell degranulation and leukocyte activation. Neurotransmitters, released peripherally from injured tissues, blood cells (platelets, white cells, macrophages, lymphocytes, mast cells) and free endings of afferent fibres (by axon reflex), are numerous, hence the use of the

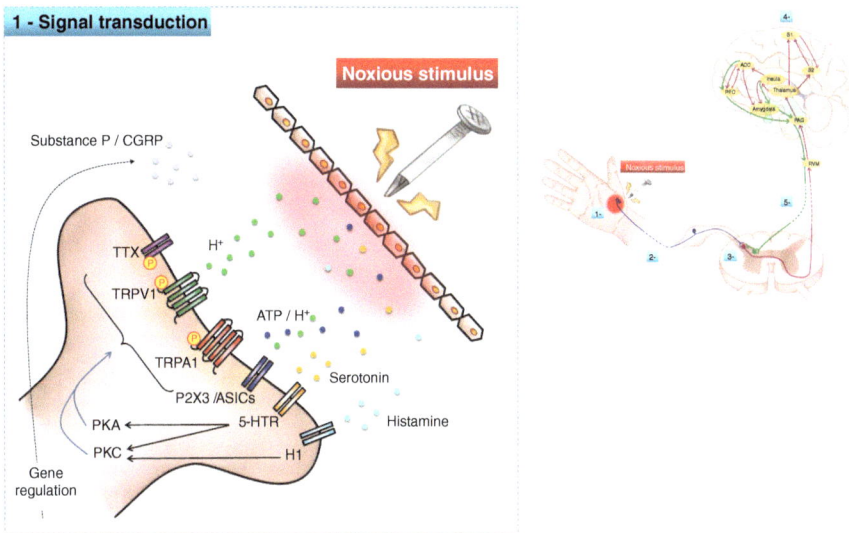

Fig. 2.3 Transduction of pain signal at peripheral site following noxious stimulus (*5-HTR* serotonin receptor, *ATP* adenosine triphosphate, *CGRP* calcitonin gene-related peptide, *H⁺* ion hydrogen, *H1* histamine receptor, *PKA* protein kinase A, *PKC* protein kinase C, *TRP* transient receptor potential cation channel, *TTX* voltage-gated sodium channel)

term "inflammatory soup". Among them are H^+ ions and ATP from tissue lesions, bradykinin (one of the most powerful algogenic substances), substance P and CGRP (calcitonin gene-related peptide) which are released by the free endings of nociceptors and, finally, serotonin and histamine which are released by the degranulation of mast cells. These substances act either directly on the ion channels or indirectly via the initiation of an intracellular signalling cascade involving kinases resulting mainly in phosphorylation of TRP and voltage-gated sodium (TTX) channels (Ji et al. 2003; Le Bars and Adam 2002). In response to a stimulus, TRP and TTX channels induce an inward cation current, mainly calcium (Ca^{2+}) and sodium (Na^+) ions, that causes cell depolarization and release of neuropeptides at the peripheral and central sites (Fig. 2.3).

Thus, the release of the actors of this inflammatory soup results in sensitization of nociceptors which then respond excessively to nociceptive stimulation (phenomenon of hyperalgesia) or which respond to normally non-painful stimuli (phenomenon of allodynia).

2.2.2 Central Mechanisms: Spinal Level

All primary sensory receptors establish synaptic connections with neurons of dorsal horn (grey matter) of the spinal cord. These second neurons project their axons and transmit the nociceptive message to higher brain areas (supraspinal sites).

2.2.2.1 Primary Afferent Fibre Input

Upon arrival in the radiculomedullary junction (at the entrance to the dorsal root of the spinal cord), the sensory fibres split according to their type and the location of their arrival in the spinal cord. The grey matter of the spinal cord has a laminar configuration composed of columns of neurons. These layers (laminae) of neurons are distinguished according to the Rexed classification (Rexed 1952). The C-fibres project mainly in the surface of laminae I and II, and the Aδ-fibres project into laminae I and V, while the Aβ-fibres relay tactile information into the deeper laminae III, IV and V and up to the ventral horn of the spinal cord to establish connections with the motor neurons responsible for the withdrawal reflex during painful stimulation (Basbaum et al. 2009). It is within these laminae that the first central relay of the nociceptive inputs between the primary afferent fibres and the second-order spinal neurons takes place.

2.2.2.2 Spinal Sensory Neurons

The central relay of nociceptive information involves two types of spinal sensory neurons that can also be found at thalamic and cortical sites:

(a) Nociceptive-specific neurons are excited only by painful stimuli, and their cell bodies are mainly located in the superficial laminae I and II and, to a lesser extent, in laminae V, VI, VII and X. They respond to high-intensity stimuli, sufficiently intense to cause injury, transmitted by afferent Aδ- and C-fibres of various origins (cutaneous, articular, visceral) (Schmidt and Willis 2007).
(b) Nociceptive non-specific neurons, called wide dynamic range (WDR) neurons or polymodal sensory neurons, respond to both noxious (Aδ- and C-fibres) and innocuous stimuli (Aα,β-fibres). Their cell bodies are mainly located deeper in lamina V and, to a lesser extent, in laminae I and II. The activity of these neurons is proportional to the intensity of the stimulation. One WDR neuron can receive both noxious and innocuous inputs (Schmidt and Willis 2007).

In parallel with this classification taking into account the sensitivity of spinal neurons to the sensory information coming from the primary afferent fibres, spinal neurons of the dorsal horn can be classified according to their extramedullary (projection neurons) or intramedullary targets (spinal interneurons).

(a) The projection neuron axons are grouped into ascending medullary tracts relaying the nociceptive input to the supraspinal sites. These neurons respond to nociceptive inputs and can be assimilated to nociceptive-specific and/or WDR neurons (Doyle and Hunt 1999; Mantyh et al. 1997).
(b) Spinal interneurons project their axons only into the dorsal horn of the spinal cord and are activated by nociceptive inputs from the primary afferent fibres. Two types of interneurons are identified according to their excitatory or inhibitory action at the postsynaptic level. Excitatory interneurons may indirectly activate projection neurons in the superficial and deeper laminae and may exert excitatory feedback on the primary afferent fibres, amplifying their signal (Basbaum et al. 2009; Neumann et al. 2008). Conversely, inhibitory interneu-

rons limit the transmission of nociceptive inputs by directly acting on projection neurons and/or spinal endings of the nociceptive primary afferent fibres.

2.2.2.3 Neurotransmitters

Following nociceptive stimulation, the action potential generated by the ionotropic receptors located on the periphery of the nociceptor (TRP, TTX channels) is transmitted along the axon to induce the release of neurotransmitters at the spinal level. Two types of neurotransmitters are involved in the transmission and modulation of nociceptive information: excitatory neurotransmitters such as glutamate and aspartate (generating a rapid excitatory postsynaptic potential (EPSP) in ascending projection neurons) and inhibitory neurotransmitters such as glycine or GABA (generating inhibitory postsynaptic potential, IPSP). Afferent nociceptive fibres (especially C-fibres) also release many neuropeptides such as substance P, neurotensin, vasoactive intestinal peptide (VIP), CGRP and cholecystokinin (CCK), inducing slow EPSP, in ascending projection neurons. Neurotransmitters, released from vesicles by the primary afferent fibre (or presynaptic neuron) in the synaptic cleft, enable the transmission of nociceptive signals to the second-order neurons (postsynaptic neurons). The postsynaptic membrane is not excitable electrically, but chemically. These molecules, therefore, bind to their specific receptors on the postsynaptic membrane and induce depolarization of the target neuron and a generation of an action potential. This action potential enables the transduction of the nociceptive input and its transmission to the supraspinal sites.

2.2.3 Central Mechanisms: Supraspinal Level

Convergent neuron axons of the dorsal horn of the spinal cord (laminae I and V), carrying nociceptive and non-nociceptive information, constitute the ascending medullary tracts that transmit the information to different supraspinal sites. The majority of these axons decussate at the level of the medullary segment to terminate their path in the thalamus, leaving some fibres in the rostral-ventromedial medulla (RVM) and the periaqueductal grey matter (PAG) (Fig. 2.1) (Bernard and Villanueva 2009; Todd 2002). Connections between the PAG and the RVM involve descending inhibitory systems that regulate nerve impulses that originate from the spinal cord. Among the brain areas that manage sensory and nociceptive information, the S1 somatosensory cortex treats the nociceptive input as tactile information, and the S2 distinguishes high-intensity and potentially dangerous inputs. These brain areas are involved in the location, quality, intensity and duration of pain sensations. Some WDR neurons project into anterior insular and cingulate cortices. The amygdala also seems to receive information from nociceptive-specific neurons of lamina I. These structures participate in emotional integration (aversive characteristic of painful experience), memory and behavioural adaptation (Almeida et al. 2004; Basbaum et al. 2009; Calvino 2006).

2.2.4   When Acute Pain Becomes Chronic

Under normal conditions, painful sensation mediated by noxious stimulation decreases with the progression of healing of the injury. However, intense and persistent injury, or disease-mediated pain, can activate secondary mechanisms in the peripheral and central nervous systems and can lead to allodynia and hyperalgesia. One of the essential processes involved in the development and maintenance of chronic pain is the sensitization of the nociceptive system that occurs following repetitive or particularly intense noxious stimuli. This sensitization involves a decrease in activation thresholds of the nociceptive system, inducing amplification of the response to subsequent stimuli. The molecular and cellular pathophysiological mechanisms involved in the triggering and maintenance of chronic pain are very complex and occur at both peripheral and central level (Gangadharan and Kuner 2013).

2.2.5   Peripheral Sensitization

Peripheral sensitization refers to an increase in sensitivity of nociceptive primary afferent fibres to nociceptive stimuli and algogenic substances and causes primary and secondary hyperalgesia. Under physiological pain conditions, this sensitization is limited in time and plays a role in the protection of the body. In chronic and neuropathic pain states, this phenomenon partly becomes the cause of the persistence of pain (Basbaum et al. 2009).

At the origin of this peripheral sensitization lies the phenomenon of inflammation which initially recruits non-neuronal cells (macrophages, mast cells, platelets, keratinocytes, endothelial cells and fibroblasts) and then neuronal cells able to release the "inflammatory soup" comprised of pro-inflammatory and pro-algesic molecules. These molecules modify the intrinsic properties of nociceptive primary afferent fibres by intracellular transduction mechanisms involved in modulation of TRP receptor channel sensitivity (Bautista et al. 2006; Kwan et al. 2006). Under these conditions, the nociceptors' activation threshold is lowered, and the excitability of primary afferent fibres is increased. These fibres are also capable of spontaneously discharging action potentials in the absence of any external stimulation.

2.2.6   Central Sensitization

Although central sensitization is closely linked to peripheral sensitization, it differs in terms of molecular mechanisms and manifestations. Central sensitization involves low-threshold mechanoreceptors (which do not lead to pain under normal physiological conditions), turning Aβ-fibres into nociceptive fibres (Latremoliere and Woolf 2009; Woolf and Salter 2000). It also induces pain hypersensitivity in non-inflamed tissues by altering the sensory response to normal impulses.

When neurons of the dorsal horn of the spinal cord are subjected to central sensitization, their hyperexcitability may result in a development of spontaneous activity, an increase in their response to supraliminal stimuli, a decrease in their activation threshold and an increase in their receptive field. Several features are specific to central sensitization, including conversion of nociceptive-specific neurons to WDR neurons, responding to both non-noxious and nociceptive stimuli or even progressive increases in neuron response during repetitive identical stimuli on the same territory (Latremoliere and Woolf 2009).

This central sensitization takes place at the level of dorsal horn laminae I and V neurons and in some brain structures such as the thalamus, amygdala and anterior cingulate cortex (ACC). Using functional magnetic resonance imaging (fMRI) or positron emission tomography (PET) techniques, new structures have been implicated such as the parabrachial nucleus, and PAG (Peyron et al. 2000; Shih et al. 2008). Central sensitization is divided in two phases: an induction phase and a maintenance phase that are described below (Ji et al. 2003; Latremoliere and Woolf 2009).

2.2.6.1 Induction Phase of Central Sensitization

The continuous release of glutamate, substance P and CGRP by the primary nociceptive afferent fibres following inflammatory or nerve injury induces the activation of their specific postsynaptic receptors, causing an increase in the excitability of the nociceptive neurons of the dorsal horn of the spinal cord. Glutamate binds to the ionotropic receptors α-amino-3-hydroxy-5-methyl-4-isoxazolepropionic acid (AMPA), N-methyl-D-aspartate (NMDA) and kainate (KA) and several metabotropic glutamate receptors (mGluRs). This binding to these receptors leads to hyperexcitability of the spinal postsynaptic neurons due to the entry of Ca^{2+} which is responsible for the activation of cellular signalling proteins such as calcium-calmodulin (that activate calcium-calmodulin kinase II (CaMKII)), protein kinase C (PKC) and protein kinase A (PKA). The release of substance P, CGRP and brain-derived neurotrophic factor (BDNF) also contributes to the activation of several intracellular signalling pathways such as the extracellular signal-regulated protein kinase (ERK), phosphorylation of cAMP response element binding protein (CREB) and the activation of phospholipase C (PLC) and PKC (Pezet 2014; Pezet et al. 2002). In clinical practice a number of NMDA receptor antagonists (ketamine, memantine, dextromethorphan) have been shown to inhibit the hyperexcitability of spinal cord nociceptive neurons and may decrease neuropathic pain intensity (Collins et al. 2010; Zhou et al. 2011). Finally, pro-inflammatory bradykinin, via its binding to the B2 receptor, activates the PKC, PKA and ERK pathways (Latremoliere and Woolf 2009).

2.2.6.2 Maintaining Central Sensitization

Central sensitization is maintained by a number of modulators including ERK protein kinase. It enters in the spinal neuron nucleus and lead to CREB phosphorylation and Elk-1 activation. Both proteins induce gene transcription for long-term synaptic enhancement (Ji et al. 2003; Latremoliere and Woolf 2009). This mechanism leads to an increase in synaptic transmission in the dorsal horn of the spinal cord and contributes to the development of pathological nociceptive response by increasing NMDA receptor activity (by post-translational phosphorylation) and by increasing the number of NMDA and AMPA receptors at the synaptic level (Ji et al. 2003; Latremoliere and Woolf 2009; Petrenko et al. 2003).

2.3   Neuropathic Pain

Neuropathic pain is a specific chronic pain state defined in 2008 by the International Association for the Study of Pain (IASP) as "pain arising as a direct consequence of a lesion or disease affecting the somatosensory system" (Finnerup et al. 2016). Although the origin and intensity of pain may vary from one individual to another, neuropathic pain has specific common characteristics. Patients typically experience paradoxical pain sensory perceptions as hypersensitivity ("positive signs") combined with reduced sensitivity ("negative" signs). "Positive" signs result in spontaneous sensations or pains (not induced by a stimulus) such as:

- Transient and spontaneous paroxysmal pain, similar to electric shock or stabbing
- Superficial pain, related to continuous pain often described as burning sensations
- Paraesthesia, representing several unpleasant symptoms that are not painful, such as tingling, pins and needles, numbness, itching

Many patients also experience evoked pain, that is, pain caused by a stimulus. Patients usually experience mechanical (dynamic and/or static) and thermal (hot and/or cold) allodynia or hyperalgesia.

The data currently available can help to understand the links between neuropathic symptoms and the underlying pathophysiological mechanisms (Klein et al. 2005).

In neuropathic pain conditions, the increase of TTXr channels and TRPV1 receptor expression on peripheral free nerve endings causes a rise in the excitation and spontaneous excitability of these neurons after axonal injury due to the importance of the sodium channels in the genesis of the action potential (Zimmermann 2001). Furthermore, the nociceptive afferent C-fibres overexpress the $\alpha 2\delta$ calcium channel subunit involved in the kinetics of activation and inactivation of the channel and in the regulation of the Ca^{2+} current amplitude. Thus, the increase in Ca^{2+} entry into the primary afferent fibre plays an important role in the release of neurotransmitters at the dorsal horn of the spinal cord and at the level of the peripheral free nerve endings (Nieto-Rostro et al. 2014). In clinical practice, anticonvulsants are used in neuropathic pain management, and their analgesic effect is mediated by the inhibition of the $\alpha 2\delta$ calcium channel subunit, causing a decrease in central sensitization and in transmission of the nociceptive information (Patel and Dickenson 2016).

2.4   Pain Modulation Mechanisms

Several physiological processes, mainly the descending pain modulatory circuits, are at play in pain. In the case of acute pain, modulatory systems are activated to modulate pain sensation by decreasing nociceptive input transmission and integration (Purves et al. 2001). In chronic pain states, however, several studies have suggested that there is a dysfunction in these descending control systems that is involved in pain "chronicization" (Ossipov et al. 2014). In elderly people, many of the following pain modulation mechanisms may also be altered, causing an alteration in pain perception and pain reports.

2.5   Opioidergic System

Transmission of nociceptive information can be modulated by endogenous peptides, endorphins that mimic the effects of morphine by binding to opiate receptors. There are three main families of endorphins: (1) the proenkephalin at the origin of enkephalins, (2) the pro-opiomelanocortin precursor of beta-endorphin and (3) the prodynorphin at the origin of dynorphins and neoendorphins (Kieffer and Gavériaux-Ruff 2002). These endogenous opioids are among the key mediators involved in descending inhibitory controls and are released at various locations in the peripheral and central nervous systems (Budai and Fields 1998; Lesniak and Lipkowski 2011). There are three classes of pre- and postsynaptic opioid receptors, μ (MOR), δ (DOR) and κ (KOR), expressed at both central and peripheral levels. Endogenous opioid binding results in a decrease in the release of pro-algesic mediators such as substance P and CGRP and in a reduction of nociceptor excitability (Lesniak and Lipkowski 2011).

2.6   Descending Inhibitory Controls from the Brainstem

Inhibitory controls descending towards the spinal cord are mainly performed by the PAG (mesencephalic structure that sends projections on the RVM, the *locus coeruleus* and the *locus sub-coeruleus*) and the RVM (bulbar region) which connect the NRM and the paragigantocellular nucleus. The neurons of these structures, involved in the blockade of nociceptive inputs, are serotoninergic neurons. The axons of these neurons, derived from RVM (notably NRM), project directly onto nociceptive non-specific neurons of the dorsal horn of the spinal cord at different spinal segments. In addition, these descending inhibitory controls also involve noradrenergic neurons from the *locus coeruleus* and the *locus sub-coeruleus* (Ossipov et al. 2014). The axons of these neurons release norepinephrine at laminae II and V of the dorsal horn, capable of binding to α2-noradrenergic receptors (Calvino and Grilo 2006).

2.7   Diffuse Noxious Inhibitory Controls Induced by Nociceptive Stimulation (DNICs)

DNICs are phenomena in which all nociceptive non-specific neurons of the dorsal horn of the spinal cord are strongly inhibited by nociceptive stimulation applied to parts of the body different from the initial pain site (heterotopic stimulation). DNICs may result from central activation at the brainstem, particularly involving the *subnucleus reticularis dorsalis* (SRD) belonging to the bulbar reticular formation (Le Bars et al. 1992). The neurotransmitters involved in this pain control system are endorphins and serotonin. The clinical importance of assessing the integrity of DNICs is based on the fact that DNIC-mediated pain inhibition is reduced in many cases of chronic pain (Arendt-Nielsen et al. 2010; Kosek and Ordeberg 2000; Lautenbacher and Rollman 1997; Pickering et al. 2014; Pielsticker et al. 2005; Sandrini et al. 2006). These descending inhibitory controls are enhanced, in clinical practice, with the use of antidepressants whose analgesic properties are mediated by their potency to inhibit the reuptake of monoamines (tricyclic), serotonin and noradrenaline (SNRIs) (Artigas et al. 2002; Gilron et al. 2015).

2.8   Descending Facilitatory Controls

Descending facilitatory controls from the brainstem, and particularly RVM, can intensify nociceptive stimulation in the spinal cord. Fields and colleagues (Fields 1992) identified three families of cells in rats:

1. "ON" cells, whose activation facilitates the transmission of the nociceptive input at the converging neurons of the dorsal horn of the spinal cord
2. "OFF" cells whose activation may strengthen the descending inhibition of the nociceptive spinal message
3. "Neutral" cells that do not respond to nociceptive stimuli

These "ON/OFF" cells are differentially recruited by the supraspinal structures involved in fear, disease and psychological stress to enhance or inhibit pain. Dynamic changes in the balance between pain inhibition and pain facilitation mediated by brainstem structures are likely to contribute to pathological pain states (Heinricher et al. 2009).

2.9   Age Differences in Clinical Pain States

With ageing, sensory signals are slower and fainter, and the warning system of pain may become less effective. In addition to the disruption of the equilibrium between facilitatory and inhibitory pathways, other factors such as depression, cognitive impairment, past pain experience, altered body image and social isolation complicate the clinical pain presentation in older people. In clinical settings, practitioners are required to care for a group composed of healthy community-dwelling persons and frail "oldest old" individuals with heterogeneous health statuses (Pickering 2005).

Acute pain, particularly that of visceral origin, has often been the focus of the literature to illustrate age differences. Conditions associated with visceral pain such as myocardial infarction, renal disease, gallstones, and pleuritic pain involve vital functions and play a large part in the morbidity and the mortality of older people.

Another complexity of the process of visceral pain initiation and transmission is that it is often poorly localized (often referred to other locations) and is not always linked to tissue injury (Raja 1999), making its diagnosis even more difficult in older people (Pickering 2005). Absence or decrease of abdominal pain is more described in older patients compared with younger adults particularly in the case of ulcer disease (Clinch et al. 1984; Hilton et al. 2001), appendicitis and peritonitis (Albano et al. 1975) and pancreatitis (Lankisch et al. 1991; Wilson and Imrie 1988). Compared with younger adults, in the elderly atypical acute pain presentation and lower intensity of pain also concern cardiac pain (Tresch 1996), pulmonary disease (Liston et al. 1994; Timmons et al. 2003) and oral pain (Pau et al. 2003).

Chronic pain affects 25–80% of older people (Pereira et al. 2014) and is greater in advanced age (Rustøen et al. 2005), particularly in musculoskeletal disease, arthritis, burning mouth syndrome and neuropathic pain states (Pickering 2005). However, studies have shown that prevalence of pain complaints peaks at middle age and decreases in older persons (Andersson et al. 1993; Cook et al. 1989; Gagliese and Melzack 1999; Lipton et al. 1993; Wright et al. 1995) notably in migraine, temporomandibular pain and facial pain (Pickering 2005). In addition, the prevalence of pain that interferes with everyday life increases incrementally with age (Thomas et al. 2004) probably because osteoarthritis dominates the pain pattern in older adults and because comorbidity amplifies the level of restricted activity (Pickering 2005).

2.9.1   Changes in Pain Perception and Pain Thresholds with Ageing

2.9.1.1 Changes of Clinical Pain Report in Older Age

Clinical pain reports in older adults (mainly uncontrolled studies) reveal that pain may be much less frequent and severe in a variety of somatic and visceral medical conditions, including myocardial ischemia, pneumonia, appendicitis, peptic ulcer, post-operative pain and cancer (Pickering 2005). The severity of chest pain is also less after controlling for severity of myocardial ischemia (Rittger et al. 2011). A retrospective review of more than 1500 cases of various types of malignancy revealed similar age differences in the incidence of pain between younger adults and older adults (55% versus 26% with pain) (Cherng et al. 1991) and a decline in reported pain severity (Caraceni and Portenoy 1999). In the post-operative recovery period, older adults have been shown to display a 10–20% reduction in pain intensity for each additional decade of life after 60 years, even after controlling for the extent of operative tissue damage (Thomas et al. 1998). The prevalence of radiographic osteoarthritis steadily increases until at least 90 years of age and, undoubtedly, contributes to much of the pain seen in older people. However, the report of arthritic pain severity does not show the same ageing trend. After accounting for disease severity, the intensity of arthritic pain has been reported to decrease (Parker et al. 1988), increase (Chiou et al. 2009) or remain unchanged with advancing age (Gagliese and Melzack 1997). Given that the studies cited above are essentially uncontrolled clinical case reports, it is impossible to determine whether any observed decline in pain reflects actual age differences in the pain experience or differences in disease severity and/or the willingness to report pain as a symptom. Nonetheless, based on the available evidence, it does appear that advancing age is often associated with reduced severity of pain as well as reduced frequency of pain as a presenting symptom, and this has important implications for clinical diagnosis and management. There are a variety of potential reasons that atypical pain presentations are more common in older people, including the presence of comorbidity, altered beliefs about pain and age-related changes in physiological functions, including within the nociceptive system itself.

2.9.1.2 Importance of Psychosocial Factors on Pain Perception in Older Age

With advanced age, some psychosocial factors such as beliefs, symptom meaning and fear can alter the perceptual pain experience and consequent level of suffering (Gibson 2005). Pain is often associated with a threat of illness, signifying function and independence loss and, sometimes, death. However, compared to younger adults, older people do not perceive all pain as a major stressor responsible for altered health status. In fact, studies show that pain is not inevitably related to interference in daily life activities (Thomas et al. 2004) and physical impairment and may be related to high self-rated health status (Collerton et al. 2009). It is conceivable that older people suffering from pain can be perceived to have aged successfully (Collis and Waterfield 2015; Reichstadt et al. 2007; Young et al. 2009). The reason explaining this lack of relationship between pain symptoms and self-ratings of health in elderly persons is their understanding that health status is dynamic and can normally decrease with age (Ebrahimi et al. 2012). In fact, older people perceive pain as a natural process associated with increased age, and this can lead to pain acceptance and lack of interest in finding appropriate treatment (Collis and Waterfield 2015; Gignac et al. 2006; Grime et al. 2010). Other changes of pain attitudes and beliefs in older persons concern age-related increase in stoicism and cautiousness to consider a sensation as painful (Gibson 2005; Yong et al. 2003). Thus, stoic attitudes are implicated in the under-reporting of pain symptoms in older people (Abdulla et al. 2013). These changes in psychosocial factors regarding beliefs and misattribution of pain symptoms to the physiological ageing process may be linked with an alteration of pain perception and decrease in the importance placed on aches and pains as an alarm signal, reducing the capacity of the healthcare practitioner to provide the appropriate pain management.

2.9.2   Changes of Pathophysiology of Pain in Older Age

The lengthening of life expectancy is associated with the development of multiple long-term illnesses affecting nearly 65% of population aged 65 and older. Long-term neurological conditions result from injury or disease of the nervous system that will affect individuals for the rest of their life. This can cause a range of different problems for the individual including worsening mobility, sensory problems such as loss of vision or hearing, pain and altered sensation, dementia or cognitive/behavioural impairment and communication disorders, inducing difficulties in speaking and in fully understanding what is said or written (Turner-Stokes et al. 2008).

Pain management is a major concern in older people, but remains insufficient either at home, in nursing homes or in hospital care (Boerlage et al. 2008; Gibson and Lussier 2012; Mehta et al. 2010; Miró et al. 2007). The peripheral and central nervous systems are both affected by the progressive loss of neurons and nerve fibres caused by age-related disorders. Functional, structural and biochemical changes have been reported in the peripheral nerves of older people. With advancing age, studies have shown a reduction in the density of unmyelinated and myelinated fibres with signs of damage or degeneration inducing a marked decrease of peripheral nerve conduction velocity (Drac et al. 1991; Verdú et al. 2000). Age-related changes in pain thresholds are contradictory across studies, but a meta-analysis (Gibson and Farrell 2004) including 40 studies of nociceptive electrical, mechanical and thermal stimulations showed that pain threshold increases with age, meaning that older people are less sensitive to moderate pain. These findings are consistent with severe and persistent pain prevalence in the elderly experiencing lower pain thresholds, indicating impairment in the early warning functions of pain and a decrease in the pain complaints, contributing to a higher risk of late diagnosis of trauma or illness (abdominal pain, myocardial infarction, pulmonary embolism, etc.) (Edwards 2005; Gibson and Farrell 2004; Pickering 2005).

These changes in pain perception can be attributed to alterations in structure (axonal involution and decreased myelin), neurochemistry (with reduced levels in substance P, CGRP and somatostatin at spinal and supraspinal levels) and function of both the peripheral and central nervous systems, including neurochemical degradation in opioidergic and serotonergic systems (Banerjee and Poddar 2016; Bergman et al. 1996; Gagliese and Farrell 2005; Helme and McKernan 1985; Hukkanen et al. 2002; Li and Duckles 1993). There is also a decline in NMDA receptor expression and density (Magnusson et al. 2010; Piggott et al. 1992), and, in supraspinal sites, a reduction in synthesis and binding of some neurotransmitters such as GABA, norepinephrine, dopamine, glutamate, acetylcholine and opioids has been observed (Amenta et al. 1991; Barili et al. 1998). The endogenous pain inhibitory system, which originates in the brainstem and exerts an antinociceptive effect via opioid and serotonergic systems at the spinal level, is altered during ageing (Hamm and Knisely 1985, 1986; Riley et al. 2010). In several studies, ageing was also associated with a reduction in the mechanisms of DNIC response in comparison with healthy younger adults (Edwards 2005; Kosek and Ordeberg 2000; Lariviere et al. 2007). This alteration may reduce the ability of older people to manage severe pain, resulting in a prolonged pain state and vulnerability. Changes in brain areas involved in the integration and interpretation of pain sensations may occur during ageing, but such pain processing is not well described. However, one study suggested that pain perception during normal ageing is associated with functional, rather than structural, alterations in pain processing areas, particularly in the insular and somatosensory cortices at S1 (Fig. 2.4).

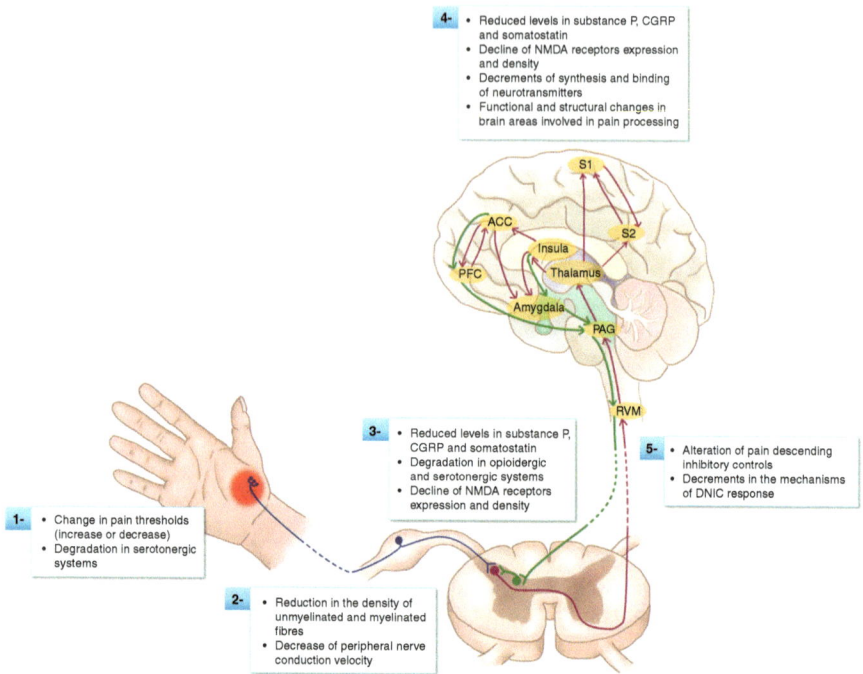

Fig. 2.4 Pathophysiological changes of pain processing in elderly people

In addition to pathophysiological factors, cognitive state is decisive in pain perception. Impairment or loss of functions, such as attention, concentration, alertness, memory during ageing and neurodegenerative disorders that often accompany ageing, tend to diminish complaint of pain or bias the interpretation of pain cues of demented patients (Achterberg et al. 2013; Pieper et al. 2013).

2.9.2.1 Changes of Central Nervous System in Older Age: The Impact of Dementia

With advancing age, many changes take place in the central nervous system, resulting in pain processing modifications. Studies of the human brain revealed a small loss of neurons and decreased brain volume that was most pronounced in the prefrontal cortex and hippocampus and less pronounced in the midbrain and brainstem regions (Edwards 2005; Farrell 2012). Neuronal losses, contributing to the reduction in grey matter volume, result in shrinking of neurons, loss of synaptic spines and decrease in dendritic synapses of existing neurons (Dickstein et al. 2007; Farrell 2012; Peters and Rosene 2003).

Ageing also coincides with a greater risk for dementia. As people with dementia become less communicative, pain assessment and subsequent pain management may be more difficult in this frail population. Scherder argued that neuropathology affecting the brain neuronal system involved in pain processing will strengthen the reliability of pain assessment and may reduce or prevent undertreatment of pain in these patients (Scherder 2017). Across several studies, Scherder and coworkers showed that pain processing alterations may differ between various subtypes of neuropathologies such as Alzheimer's disease (AD), frontotemporal dementia, subcortical vascular dementia, multiple sclerosis or Parkinson's disease (Binnekade et al. 2017; Scherder et al. 2005). The pain processing systems affected by these alterations are the medial and lateral pain systems. For a comprehensive description of these both systems, see Scherder et al. (2003).

In AD, most of the areas of the medial pain system undergo degeneration, including the amygdala and hippocampus, resulting in a decline in memory of pain. Additionally, atrophy of the locus coeruleus, ACC, amygdala, hippocampus and S2 are responsible for a deterioration in cognitive/evaluative aspects of persistent pain that is prevalent in older people in nursing home setting (Helme and Gibson 2001; Scherder 2017). The transmission of nociceptive information to S1 is not disrupted, and this may explain why, in some studies, pain threshold in patients with AD is no different to the pain threshold of patients without AD (Defrin et al. 2015). These findings should not lead us to conclude that the decrease in the motivational/affective aspects of pain in patients with AD diminished their pain suffering compared with patients without AD (Scherder 2017). In fact, a study performed by Cole and coworkers showed that applying nociceptive mechanical stimuli to patients with AD showed that both medial and lateral pain system activities were not affected (Cole et al. 2006).

In vascular dementia, subcortical white matter lesions (Barber et al. 1999) result in a deafferentation of pain between the cortical and subcortical areas (Farrell et al. 1996; Mori 2002) explaining that patients with lower global cognitive functioning may more suffer from pain (Scherder et al. 2015).

Studies have shown that patients with frontal frontotemporal dementia have higher pain thresholds and may suffer from less pain than patients without frontotemporal dementia or other types of dementia (Bathgate et al. 2001; Carlino et al. 2010). These results might be explained by a decline in cerebral blood flow to the ACC and the prefrontal cortex (Varrone et al. 2002), both areas playing an important role in the motivational/affective pain processing (Scherder 2017).

Although several studies have been conducted on the subject, more experimental and clinical studies are needed to study the influence of the various subtypes of dementia on pain processing (Scherder 2017).

2.10 Summary

- With ageing, many biopsychosocial and pathophysiological changes are responsible for under-reporting of pain compared to younger adults.
- Beliefs and attitudes towards pain symptoms thought to be inevitably associated with increased age induce acceptance and stoicism that may be responsible for undertreatment of pain.
- Age-related pathophysiological pain changes more frequently reported are increase in pain threshold and decrease in density and conduction velocity of nociceptive fibres.

- Ageing is related to neurochemical (notably degradation of opioidergic and serotoninergic systems, reduction in algogenic substances) and pharmacodynamic changes (decrease in NMDA receptor expression and in neurotransmitter binding).
- Alteration of descending inhibitory controls are frequently reported in older adults compared to their younger counterparts.
- Structural and functional alterations in the brain areas responsible for pain processing may modify pain perception of older people, especially those with various types of dementia.

References

Abdulla A, Adams N, Bone M, Elliott AM, Gaffin J, Jones D, et al. Guidance on the management of pain in older people. Age Ageing. 2013;42(Suppl 1):i1–57.

Achterberg WP, Pieper MJ, van Dalen-Kok AH, de Waal MW, Husebo BS, Lautenbacher S, et al. Pain management in patients with dementia. Clin Interv Aging. 2013;8:1471–82.

Albano WA, Zielinski CM, Organ CH. Is appendicitis in the aged really different? Geriatrics. 1975;30(1 Sz):81–8.

Almeida TF, Roizenblatt S, Tufik S. Afferent pain pathways: a neuroanatomical review. Brain Res. 2004;1000(1–2):40–56.

Amenta F, Zaccheo D, Collier WL. Neurotransmitters, neuroreceptors and aging. Mech Ageing Dev. 1991;61(3):249–73.

Andersson HI, Ejlertsson G, Leden I, Rosenberg C. Chronic pain in a geographically defined general population: studies of differences in age, gender, social class, and pain localization. Clin J Pain. 1993;9(3):174–82.

Arendt-Nielsen L, Nie H, Laursen MB, Laursen BS, Madeleine P, Simonsen OH, et al. Sensitization in patients with painful knee osteoarthritis. Pain. 2010;149(3):573–81.

Artigas F, Nutt DJ, Shelton R. Mechanism of action of antidepressants. Psychopharmacol Bull. 2002;36(Suppl 2):123–32.

Banerjee S, Poddar MK. Aging-induced changes in brain regional serotonin receptor binding: effect of Carnosine. Neuroscience. 2016;319:79–91.

Barber R, Scheltens P, Gholkar A, Ballard C, McKeith I, Ince P, et al. White matter lesions on magnetic resonance imaging in dementia with Lewy bodies, Alzheimer's disease, vascular dementia, and normal aging. J Neurol Neurosurg Psychiatry. 1999;67(1):66–72.

Barili P, De Carolis G, Zaccheo D, Amenta F. Sensitivity to ageing of the limbic dopaminergic system: a review. Mech Ageing Dev. 1998;106(1–2):57–92.

Basbaum AI, Bautista DM, Scherrer G, Julius D. Cellular and molecular mechanisms of pain. Cell. 2009;139(2):267–84.

Bathgate D, Snowden JS, Varma A, Blackshaw A, Neary D. Behaviour in frontotemporal dementia, Alzheimer's disease and vascular dementia. Acta Neurol Scand. 2001;103(6):367–78.

Bautista DM, Jordt S-E, Nikai T, Tsuruda PR, Read AJ, Poblete J, et al. TRPA1 mediates the inflammatory actions of environmental irritants and proalgesic agents. Cell. 2006;124(6):1269–82.

Bergman E, Johnson H, Zhang X, Hökfelt T, Ulfhake B. Neuropeptides and neurotrophin receptor mRNAs in primary sensory neurons of aged rats. J Comp Neurol. 1996;375(2):303–19.

Bernard J-F, Villanueva L. Architecture fonctionnelle des systèmes nociceptifs (Chapitre 1). In: Bouhassira D, Calvino B, editors. Douleur: physiologie, physiopathologie et pharmacologie. Dion: Arnette; 2009.

Binnekade TT, Van Kooten J, Lobbezoo F, Rhebergen D, Van der Wouden JC, Smalbrugge M, et al. Pain experience in dementia subtypes: a systematic review. Curr Alzheimer Res. 2017;14(5):471–85.

Boerlage AA, van Dijk M, Stronks DL, de Wit R, van der Rijt CCD. Pain prevalence and characteristics in three Dutch residential homes. Eur J Pain. 2008;12(7):910–6.

Budai D, Fields HL. Endogenous opioid peptides acting at mu-opioid receptors in the dorsal horn contribute to midbrain modulation of spinal nociceptive neurons. J Neurophysiol. 1998;79(2):677–87.

Calvino B. Neural basis of pain. Psychol Neuropsychiatr Vieil. 2006;4(1):7–20.

Calvino B, Grilo RM. Central pain control. Joint Bone Spine. 2006;73(1):10–6.

Caraceni A, Portenoy RK. An international survey of cancer pain characteristics and syndromes. Pain. 1999;82(3):263–74.

Carlino E, Benedetti F, Rainero I, Asteggiano G, Cappa G, Tarenzi L, et al. Pain perception and tolerance in patients with frontotemporal dementia. Pain. 2010;151(3):783–9.

Carr DB, Goudas LC. Acute pain. Lancet. 1999;353(9169):2051–8.

Cherng CH, Ho ST, Kao SJ, Ger LP. The study of cancer pain and its correlates. Ma Zui Xue Za Zhi. 1991;29(3):653–7.

Chiou A-F, Lin H-Y, Huang H-Y. Disability and pain management methods of Taiwanese arthritic older patients. J Clin Nurs. 2009;18(15):2206–16.

Clinch D, Banerjee AK, Ostick G. Absence of abdominal pain in elderly patients with peptic ulcer. Age Ageing. 1984;13(2):120–3.

Cole LJ, Farrell MJ, Duff EP, Barber JB, Egan GF, Gibson SJ. Pain sensitivity and fMRI pain-related brain activity in Alzheimer's disease. Brain. 2006;129(Pt 11):2957–65.

Collerton J, Davies K, Jagger C, Kingston A, Bond J, Eccles MP, et al. Health and disease in 85 year olds: baseline findings from the Newcastle 85+ cohort study. BMJ. 2009;339:b4904.

Collins S, Sigtermans MJ, Dahan A, Zuurmond WWA, Perez RSGM. NMDA receptor antagonists for the treatment of neuropathic pain. Pain Med. 2010;11(11):1726–42.

Collis D, Waterfield J. The understanding of pain by older adults who consider themselves to have aged successfully. Musculoskeletal Care. 2015;13(1):19–30.

Cook NR, Evans DA, Funkenstein HH, Scherr PA, Ostfeld AM, Taylor JO, et al. Correlates of headache in a population-based cohort of elderly. Arch Neurol. 1989;46(12):1338–44.

Danigo A, Magy L, Demiot C. TRPV1 dans les neuropathies douloureuses–des modèles animaux aux perspectives thérapeutiques. Med Sci (Paris). 2013;29(6–7):597–606.

Defrin R, Amanzio M, de Tommaso M, Dimova V, Filipovic S, Finn DP, et al. Experimental pain processing in individuals with cognitive impairment: current state of the science. Pain. 2015;156(8):1396–408.

Dickstein DL, Kabaso D, Rocher AB, Luebke JI, Wearne SL, Hof PR. Changes in the structural complexity of the aged brain. Aging Cell. 2007;6(3):275–84.

Doyle CA, Hunt SP. Substance P receptor (neurokinin-1)-expressing neurons in lamina I of the spinal cord encode for the intensity of noxious stimulation: a c-Fos study in rat. Neuroscience. 1999;89(1):17–28.

Drac H, Babiuch M, Wiśniewska W. Morphological and biochemical changes in peripheral nerves with aging. Neuropatol Pol. 1991;29(1–2):49–67.

Dubin AE, Patapoutian A. Nociceptors: the sensors of the pain pathway. J Clin Invest. 2010;120(11):3760–72.

Ebrahimi Z, Wilhelmson K, Moore CD, Jakobsson A. Frail elders' experiences with and perceptions of health. Qual Health Res. 2012;22(11):1513–23.

Edwards RR. Age-associated differences in pain perception and pain processing. In: Gibson SJ, Weiner DK, editors. Pain in older persons progress in pain research and management. Seattle: IASP Press; 2005. p. 45–65.

Farrell MJ. Age-related changes in the structure and function of brain regions involved in pain processing. Pain Med. 2012;13(Suppl 2):S37–43.

Farrell MJ, Katz B, Helme RD. The impact of dementia on the pain experience. Pain. 1996;67(1):7–15.

Fields HL. Is there a facilitating component to central pain modulation? APS J. 1992;1(2):71–8.

Finnerup NB, Haroutounian S, Kamerman P, Baron R, Bennett DLH, Bouhassira D, et al. Neuropathic pain: an updated grading system for research and clinical practice. Pain. 2016;157(8):1599.

Gagliese L, Farrell M. The neurobiology of aging, nociception, and pain: an integration of animal and human experimental evidence. In: Gibson SJ, Weiner DK, editors. Pain in older persons progress in pain research and management. Seattle: IASP Press; 2005. p. 25–44.

Gagliese L, Melzack R. Age differences in the quality of chronic pain: a preliminary study. Pain Res Manag. 1997;2(3):157–62.

Gagliese L, Melzack R. Age differences in the response to the formalin test in rats. Neurobiol Aging. 1999;20(6):699–707.

Gangadharan V, Kuner R. Pain hypersensitivity mechanisms at a glance. Dis Model Mech. 2013;6(4):889–95.

Gatchel RJ, Peng YB, Peters ML, Fuchs PN, Turk DC. The biopsychosocial approach to chronic pain: scientific advances and future directions. Psychol Bull. 2007;133(4):581–624.

Gibson SJ. Age differences in psychosocial aspects of pain. In: Gibson SJ, Weiner DK, editors. Pain in older persons progress in pain research and management. Seattle: IASP Press; 2005. p. 87–107.

Gibson SJ, Farrell M. A review of age differences in the neurophysiology of nociception and the perceptual experience of pain. Clin J Pain. 2004;20(4):227–39.

Gibson SJ, Lussier D. Prevalence and relevance of pain in older persons. Pain Med. 2012;13(Suppl 2):S23–6.

Gignac MAM, Davis AM, Hawker G, Wright JG, Mahomed N, Fortin PR, et al. 'What do you expect? You're just getting older': a comparison of perceived osteoarthritis-related and aging-related health experiences in middle- and older-age adults. Arthritis Rheum. 2006;55(6):905–12.

Gilron I, Baron R, Jensen T. Neuropathic pain: principles of diagnosis and treatment. Mayo Clin Proc. 2015;90(4):532–45.

Grime J, Richardson JC, Ong BN. Perceptions of joint pain and feeling well in older people who reported being healthy: a qualitative study. Br J Gen Pract. 2010;60(577):597–603.

Hamm RJ, Knisely JS. Environmentally induced analgesia: age-related decline in a neurally mediated, nonopioid system. Psychol Aging. 1986;1(3):195–201.

Hamm RJ, Knisely JS. Environmentally induced analgesia: an age-related decline in an endogenous opioid system. J Gerontol. 1985;40(3):268–74.

Heinricher MM, Tavares I, Leith JL, Lumb BM. Descending control of nociception: specificity, recruitment and plasticity. Brain Res Rev. 2009;60(1):214–25.

Helme RD, Gibson SJ. The epidemiology of pain in elderly people. Clin Geriatr Med. 2001;17(3):417–31.

Helme RD, McKernan S. Neurogenic flare responses following topical application of capsaicin in humans. Ann Neurol. 1985;18(4):505–9.

Hilton D, Iman N, Burke GJ, Moore A, O'Mara G, Signorini D, et al. Absence of abdominal pain in older persons with endoscopic ulcers: a prospective study. Am J Gastroenterol. 2001;96(2):380–4.

Hukkanen M, Platts LAM, Corbett SA, Santavirta S, Polak JM, Konttinen YT. Reciprocal age-related changes in GAP-43/B-50, substance P and calcitonin gene-related peptide (CGRP) expression in rat primary sensory neurones and their terminals in the dorsal horn of the spinal cord and subintima of the knee synovium. Neurosci Res. 2002;42(4):251–60.

IASP Task Force on Taxonomy. Classification of chronic pain: descriptions of chronic pain syndromes and definitions of pain terms. In: Merskey H, Bogduk N, editors. International association for the study of pain. 2nd ed. Seattle: IASP Press; 1994. p. 222.

IASP Taxonomy Working Group. Classification of chronic pain, 2nd ed. (Revised). Seattle: IASP Press; 2011. [cited 2018 Jan 14]. Available from: https://www.iasp-pain.org/PublicationsNews/Content.aspx?ItemNumber=1673.

Ji R-R, Kohno T, Moore KA, Woolf CJ. Central sensitization and LTP: do pain and memory share similar mechanisms? Trends Neurosci. 2003;26(12):696–705.

Kieffer BL, Gavériaux-Ruff C. Exploring the opioid system by gene knockout. Prog Neurobiol. 2002;66(5):285–306.

Klein T, Magerl W, Rolke R, Treede R-D. Human surrogate models of neuropathic pain. Pain. 2005;115(3):227–33.

Kosek E, Ordeberg G. Abnormalities of somatosensory perception in patients with painful osteoarthritis normalize following successful treatment. Eur J Pain. 2000;4(3):229–38.

Kwan KY, Allchorne AJ, Vollrath MA, Christensen AP, Zhang D-S, Woolf CJ, et al. TRPA1 contributes to cold, mechanical, and chemical nociception but is not essential for hair-cell transduction. Neuron. 2006;50(2):277–89.

Lankisch PG, Schirren CA, Kunze E. Undetected fatal acute pancreatitis: why is the disease so frequently overlooked? Am J Gastroenterol. 1991;86(3):322–6.

Larivière M, Goffaux P, Marchand S, Julien N. Changes in pain perception and descending inhibitory controls start at middle age in healthy adults. Clin J Pain. 2007;23(6):506–10.

Latremoliere A, Woolf CJ. Central sensitization: a generator of pain hypersensitivity by central neural plasticity. J Pain. 2009;10(9):895–926.

Lautenbacher S, Rollman GB. Possible deficiencies of pain modulation in fibromyalgia. Clin J Pain. 1997;13(3):189–96.

Le Bars D, Adam F. Nociceptors and mediators in acute inflammatory pain. Ann Fr Anesth Reanim. 2002;21(4):315–35.

Le Bars D, Villanueva L, Bouhassira D, Willer JC. Diffuse noxious inhibitory controls (DNIC) in animals and in man. Patol Fiziol Eksp Ter. 1992;4:55–65.

Lesniak A, Lipkowski AW. Opioid peptides in peripheral pain control. Acta Neurobiol Exp (Wars). 2011;71(1):129–38.

Li Y, Duckles SP. Effect of age on vascular content of calcitonin gene-related peptide and mesenteric vasodilator nerve activity in the rat. Eur J Pharmacol. 1993;236(3):373–8.

Lipton RB, Pfeffer D, Newman LC, Solomon S. Headaches in the elderly. J Pain Symptom Manag. 1993;8(2):87–97.

Liston R, McLoughlin R, Clinch D. Acute pneumothorax: a comparison of elderly with younger patients. Age Ageing. 1994;23(5):393–5.

Loeser JD. Concepts of pain. In: Stanton-Hicks J, Boaz R, editors. Chronic low back pain. New York: Raven Press; 1982.

Magnusson KR, Brim BL, Das SR. Selective vulnerabilities of N-methyl-D-aspartate (NMDA) receptors during brain aging. Front Aging Neurosci. 2010;2:11.

Mantyh PW, Rogers SD, Honore P, Allen BJ, Ghilardi JR, Li J, et al. Inhibition of hyperalgesia by ablation of lamina I spinal neurons expressing the substance P receptor. Science. 1997;278(5336):275–9.

McCaffery M, Beebe A. Pain: clinical manual for nursing practice. St. Louis, Missouri: C.V. Mosby; 1989.

Mehta SS, Siegler EL, Henderson CR, Reid MC. Acute pain management in hospitalized patients with cognitive impairment: a study of provider practices and treatment outcomes. Pain Med. 2010;11(10):1516–24.

Millan MJ. The induction of pain: an integrative review. Prog Neurobiol. 1999;57(1):1–164.

Miró J, Paredes S, Rull M, Queral R, Miralles R, Nieto R, et al. Pain in older adults: a prevalence study in the Mediterranean region of Catalonia. Eur J Pain. 2007;11(1):83–92.

Mori E. Impact of subcortical ischemic lesions on behavior and cognition. Ann N Y Acad Sci. 2002;977:141–8.

Nieto-Rostro M, Sandhu G, Bauer CS, Jiruska P, Jefferys JGR, Dolphin AC. Altered expression of the voltagegated calcium channel subunit α2δ -1: a comparison between two experimental models of epilepsy and a sensory nerve ligation model of neuropathic pain. Neuroscience. 2014;283:124–37.

Neumann S, Braz JM, Skinner K, Llewellyn-Smith IJ, Basbaum AI. Innocuous, not noxious, input activates PKCgamma interneurons of the spinal dorsal horn via myelinated afferent fibers. J Neurosci. 2008;28(32):7936–44.

Ossipov MH, Morimura K, Porreca F. Descending pain modulation and chronification of pain. Curr Opin Support Palliat Care. 2014;8(2):143–51.

Parker J, Frank R, Beck N, Finan M, Walker S, Hewett JE, et al. Pain in rheumatoid arthritis: relationship to demographic, medical, and psychological factors. J Rheumatol. 1988;15(3):433–7.

Patel R, Dickenson AH. Mechanisms of the gabapentinoids and α 2 δ-1 calcium channel subunit in neuropathic pain. Pharmacol Res Perspect. 2016;4(2):e00205.

Pau AKH, Croucher R, Marcenes W. Prevalence estimates and associated factors for dental pain: a review. Oral Health Prev Dent. 2003;1(3):209–20.

Pereira LV, de Vasconcelos PP, Souza LAF, de Pereira Gilberto A, Nakatani AYK, Bachion MM. Prevalence and intensity of chronic pain and self-perceived health among elderly people: a population-based study. Rev Lat Am Enfermagem. 2014;22(4):662–9.

Peters A, Rosene DL. In aging, is it gray or white? J Comp Neurol. 2003;462(2):139–43.

Petrenko AB, Yamakura T, Baba H, Shimoji K. The role of N-methyl-D-aspartate (NMDA) receptors in pain: a review. Anesth Analg. 2003;97(4):1108–16.

Peyron R, Laurent B, García-Larrea L. Functional imaging of brain responses to pain. A review and meta-analysis (2000). Neurophysiol Clin. 2000;30(5):263–88.

Pezet S. Neurotrophins and pain. Biol Aujourdhui. 2014;208(1):21–9.

Pezet S, Malcangio M, Lever IJ, Perkinton MS, Thompson SWN, Williams RJ, et al. Noxious stimulation induces Trk receptor and downstream ERK phosphorylation in spinal dorsal horn. Mol Cell Neurosci. 2002;21(4):684–95.

Pickering G. Age differences in clinical pain state. In: Gibson SJ, Weiner DK, editors. Pain in older persons progress in pain research and management. Seattle: IASP Press; 2005. p. 67–85.

Pickering G, Pereira B, Dufour E, Soule S, Dubray C. Impaired modulation of pain in patients with postherpetic neuralgia. Pain Res Manag. 2014;19(1):e19–23.

Pielsticker A, Haag G, Zaudig M, Lautenbacher S. Impairment of pain inhibition in chronic tension-type headache. Pain. 2005;118(1–2):215–23.

Pieper MJC, van Dalen-Kok AH, Francke AL, van der Steen JT, Scherder EJA, Husebø BS, et al. Interventions targeting pain or behaviour in dementia: a systematic review. Ageing Res Rev. 2013;12(4):1042–55.

Piggott MA, Perry EK, Perry RH, Court JA. [3H]MK-801 binding to the NMDA receptor complex, and its modulation in human frontal cortex during development and aging. Brain Res. 1992;588(2):277–86.

Purves D, Augustine GJ, Fitzpatrick D, Katz LC, LaMantia A-S, McNamara JO, et al. The physiological basis of pain modulation. 2nd ed. Sunderland (MA): Neuroscience; 2001.

Raja SN. Peripheral neural mechanisms of nociception. In: Melzack R, Walls PD, editors. Textbook of pain. 4th ed. London: Churchill Livingstone; 1999. p. 11–45.

Reichstadt J, Depp CA, Palinkas LA, Folsom DP, Jeste DV. Building blocks of successful aging: a focus group study of older adults' perceived contributors to successful aging. Am J Geriatr Psychiatry. 2007;15(3):194–201.

Rexed B. The cytoarchitectonic organization of the spinal cord in the cat. J Comp Neurol. 1952;96(3):414–95.

Riley JL, King CD, Wong F, Fillingim RB, Mauderli AP. Lack of Endogenous Modulation but Enhanced Decay of Prolonged Heat Pain in Older Adults. Pain. 2010;150(1):153–60.

Rittger H, Rieber J, Breithardt OA, Dücker M, Schmidt M, Abbara S, et al. Influence of age on pain perception in acute myocardial ischemia: a possible cause for delayed treatment in elderly patients. Int J Cardiol. 2011;149(1):63–7.

Rustøen T, Wahl AK, Hanestad BR, Lerdal A, Paul S, Miaskowski C. Age and the experience of chronic pain: differences in health and quality of life among younger, middle-aged, and older adults. Clin J Pain. 2005;21(6):513–23.

Sandrini G, Rossi P, Milanov I, Serrao M, Cecchini AP, Nappi G. Abnormal modulatory influence of diffuse noxious inhibitory controls in migraine and chronic tension-type headache patients. Cephalalgia. 2006;26(7):782–9.

Scherder EJA. Pain in people with dementia – its relationship to neuropathology. In: Lautenbacher S, Gibson SJ, editors. Pain in dementia. Seattle: IASP Press; 2017. p. 71–84.

Scherder EJA, Plooij B, Achterberg WP, Pieper M, Wiegersma M, Lobbezoo F, et al. Chronic pain in 'probable' vascular dementia: preliminary findings. Pain Med. 2015;16(3):442–50.

Scherder EJA, Sergeant JA, Swaab DF. Pain processing in dementia and its relation to neuropathology. Lancet Neurol. 2003;2(11):677–86.

Scherder E, Wolters E, Polman C, Sergeant J, Swaab D. Pain in Parkinson's disease and multiple sclerosis: its relation to the medial and lateral pain systems. Neurosci Biobehav Rev. 2005;29(7):1047–56.

Schmidt R, Willis W, editors. Nociceptive specific neurons. In: Encyclopedia of pain [internet]. Berlin: Springer; 2007 [cited 2018 Jan 14]. p. 1379. Available from: https://link.springer.com/referenceworkentry/10.1007/978-3-540-29805-2_2770

Shih Y-YI, Chiang Y-C, Chen J-C, Huang C-H, Chen Y-Y, Liu R-S, et al. Brain nociceptive imaging in rats using (18)f-fluorodeoxyglucose small-animal positron emission tomography. Neuroscience. 2008;155(4):1221–6.

Thomas E, Peat G, Harris L, Wilkie R, Croft PR. The prevalence of pain and pain interference in a general population of older adults: cross-sectional findings from the North Staffordshire Osteoarthritis Project (NorStOP). Pain. 2004;110(1–2):361–8.

Thomas T, Robinson C, Champion D, McKell M, Pell M. Prediction and assessment of the severity of post-operative pain and of satisfaction with management. Pain. 1998;75(2):177–85.

Timmons S, Kingston M, Hussain M, Kelly H, Liston R. Pulmonary embolism: differences in presentation between older and younger patients. Age Ageing. 2003;32(6):601–5.

Todd AJ. Anatomy of primary afferents and projection neurones in the rat spinal dorsal horn with particular emphasis on substance P and the neurokinin 1 receptor. Exp Physiol. 2002;87(2):245–9.

Tresch DD. Signs and symptoms of heart failure in elderly patients. Am J Geriatr Cardiol. 1996;5(1):27–33.

Turner-Stokes L, Sykes N, Silber E. Long-term neurological conditions: management at the interface between neurology, rehabilitation and palliative care. Clin Med. 2008;8(2):186–91.

Varrone A, Pappatà S, Caracò C, Soricelli A, Milan G, Quarantelli M, et al. Voxel-based comparison of rCBF SPET images in frontotemporal dementia and Alzheimer's disease highlights the involvement of different cortical networks. Eur J Nucl Med. 2002;29(11):1447–54.

Verdú E, Ceballos D, Vilches JJ, Navarro X. Influence of aging on peripheral nerve function and regeneration. J Peripher Nerv Syst. 2000;5(4):191–208.

Wilson C, Imrie CW. Deaths from acute pancreatitis: why do we miss the diagnosis so frequently? Int J Pancreatol. 1988;3(4):273–81.

Woolf CJ, Salter MW. Neuronal plasticity: increasing the gain in pain. Science. 2000;288(5472):1765–9.

Wright D, Barrow S, Fisher AD, Horsley SD, Jayson MI. Influence of physical, psychological and behavioural factors on consultations for back pain. Br J Rheumatol. 1995;34(2):156–61.

Yong H-H, Bell R, Workman B, Gibson SJ. Psychometric properties of the pain attitudes questionnaire (revised) in adult patients with chronic pain. Pain. 2003;104(3):673–81.

Young Y, Frick KD, Phelan EA. Can successful aging and chronic illness coexist in the same individual? A multidimensional concept of successful aging. J Am Med Dir Assoc. 2009;10(2):87–92.

Zhou H-Y, Chen S-R, Pan H-L. Targeting N-methyl-D-aspartate receptors for treatment of neuropathic pain. Expert Rev Clin Pharmacol. 2011;4(3):379–88.

Zimmermann M. Pathobiology of neuropathic pain. Eur J Pharmacol. 2001;429(1–3):23–37.

The Assessment of Pain in Older People

Thomas Fischer, Erika Sirsch, Irmela Gnass,
and Sandra Zwakhalen

Abstract

Pain assessment is a crucial step toward adequate management of pain in older adults. This chapter addresses the assessment of pain as part of a multidimensional stepwise approach. Although pain assessment uses standardized screening, assessment, and monitoring tools, it needs to be tailored to the individual patient. In the case of pain assessment in older adults, one size does not fit all is a fundamental principle. Pain is a personal and subjective experience because of numerous factors. A broad, inclusive approach to assessment is required. In this chapter several case studies highlight the differences and factors that need to be taken into account in the assessment of pain in older people.

T. Fischer
Evangelische Hochschule Dresden, University of Applied Sciences for Social Work, Education and Nursing, Dresden, Germany
e-mail: Thomas.Fischer@ehs-dresden.de

E. Sirsch
Philosophisch-Theologische Hochschule Vallendar, Vallendar, Germany
e-mail: esirsch@pthv.de

I. Gnass
Paracelsus Medical University, Institute of Nursing Science and Practice, Salzburg, Austria
e-mail: irmela.gnass@pmu.ac.at

S. Zwakhalen (✉)
Department of Health Services Research, Maastricht University, Maastricht, The Netherlands
e-mail: s.zwakhalen@maastrichtuniversity.nl

© Springer International Publishing AG, part of Springer Nature 2018
G. Pickering et al. (eds.), *Pain Management in Older Adults*, Perspectives in Nursing Management and Care for Older Adults, https://doi.org/10.1007/978-3-319-71694-7_3

3.1 Pain: A Biopsychosocial Model

The International Association for the Study of Pain (IASP) has used a biopsychosocial pain model to define pain since the 1960s, characterizing pain as a multidimensional phenomenon. According to Melzack and Wall (1996), pain consists of three dimensions: sensory-discriminatory, affective-motivational, and cognitive-evaluative. The sensory-discriminatory dimension refers to the localization of pain, the perceived pain intensity, and the sensory pain quality (how the pain feels). The affective-motivational dimension concerns, above all, emotional characteristics, how the pain is perceived emotionally, for example, whether pain is perceived as terrible, depressing, or frightening. The cognitive-evaluative dimension refers to thoughts and reflections about pain, the cause and the expected course of pain, or the estimated effect of therapy. These different pain dimensions inform the pain assessment process (Sirsch et al. 2015a).

3.2 The Assessment of Pain: A Systematic Approach

Systematic assessment must inform all stages of the pain management process. Health professionals with specific skill sets use dedicated instruments and algorithms to collect and structure information about patients and their pain experience. Pain assessment encompasses far more than just the collection of pain intensity ratings; it must be tailored to the individual patient, taking the type of pain, setting, and patient characteristics (such as age or specific conditions such as dementia) into account.

The multidimensional nature of pain, including its sensory, emotional, cognitive, and social components (Williams and Craig 2016), must be reflected in the way pain is assessed so that it can inform the management of a wide variety of pain manifestations and consequences. Pain assessment aims:

> "...to make a differential diagnosis; to predict response to treatment; to evaluate the characteristics of pain and the impact of pain on patients' lives; to assist in disability determination and establishment of limitation of physical capacity; to monitor progress following initiation of treatment; and to evaluate the effectiveness of treatment, along with the need to modify a treatment regimen, along with others.") (Turk and Melzack 2011)

Conceptually, assessment is part of the diagnostic process but separate from making an actual diagnosis (Reuschenbach 2011), but it also forms an important part of the diagnostic and clinical decision-making processes (Lipschick et al. 2009). In clinical practice, assessment and diagnostic decision-making are inextricably linked as elements of the process of care (Alfaro-LeFevre 2014).

Any type of assessment should reach beyond the use of standardized instruments and measures and always include different types of deliberate and intentional appraisals of specific phenomena or concepts such as pain. Assessment is not limited to physiological or pathophysiological aspects of a phenomenon but also extends to psychological or social aspects (Reuschenbach 2011) as well as functioning and participation (Kompetenz-Centrum Geriatrie beim Medizinischen Dienst der Krankenversicherung Nord 2009). Given the multidimensional nature of pain and the effect it may have on the lives of older adults, a broad and inclusive approach to assessment is essential.

Pain assessment in clinical practice is an ongoing process with three phases (see Fig. 3.1):

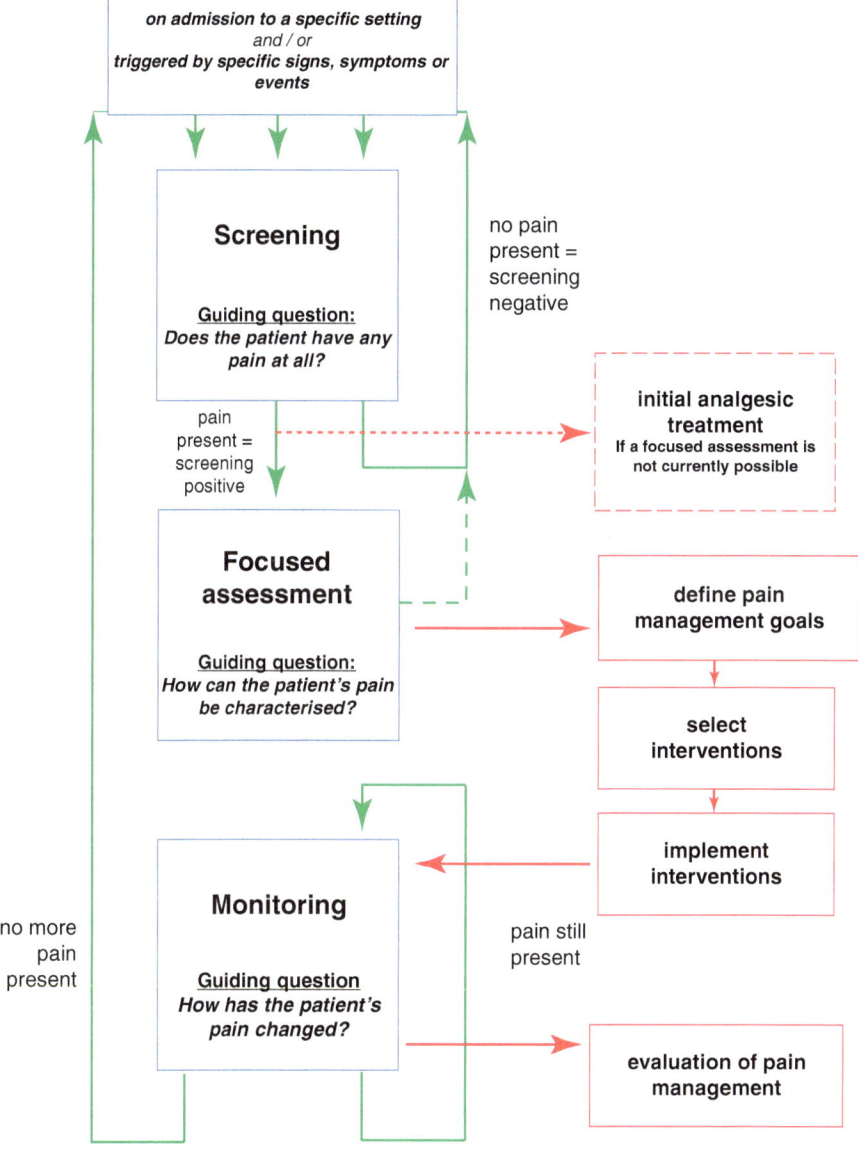

Fig. 3.1 Algorithm for pain screening, assessment, and monitoring (source: German Pain Society and DZNE 2017)

1. *Screening*: Screening is used to identify patients who are at risk of developing a particular health problem or who are already subject to a condition such as pain (Alfaro-LeFevre 2014; Wilkinson 2007). Clinical screening for pain should be guided by the question: "Does the patient have any pain at all?" If pain or pain-related problems are detected, the screening is positive, and a focused assessment of pain should follow.
2. *Focused assessment*: The aim of a focused assessment is to explore a specific health problem or condition in detail (Alfaro-LeFevre 2014; Wilkinson 2007). This should lead to a diagnosis and provides the basis for clinical decision-making regarding appropriate interventions. It also establishes a point of reference for evaluating the success of implemented interventions. A focused assessment of pain should be guided by the question: "How can this patient's pain be characterized or described?"
3. *Monitoring*: Monitoring is an ongoing process in any patient who is subject to pain and is aimed at evaluating the status of known problems and the success of implemented interventions as well as at discovering new problems that may not have been present during the initial focused assessment (Wilkinson 2012). Pain monitoring should be guided by the question: "How has the patient's pain changed?" Findings from pain monitoring may influence the choice and implementation of further interventions.

3.3 Case Descriptions of Older People and the Assessment of Pain

Within these phases nurses must take different factors into account and distinguish between the detection of chronic and acute pain (see Chap. 2). They also need to take the different needs of the older person into account and the range of problems they may experience due to physical or cognitive impairment. The following three cases illustrate these different needs in relation to pain assessment.

3.3.1 Case 1: Older Patient with Acute Pain after a Fracture

Mrs. Thomas is a 92-year-old widow who has always lived independently. Her medical history includes osteoporosis. Recently, she fractured her left hip after falling while walking in the garden. She underwent surgery and was admitted to a nursing home for rehabilitation. The physical therapist reports that Mrs. Thomas has been uncooperative. She is also unwilling to use the bathroom or go to the dining room for meals. Daily assessment of pain, using a numerical rating scale, demonstrates that she is suffering from severe pain, especially in the morning and in the evening. Her general health has deteriorated and she has, consequently, developed pressure ulcers, which has contributed even further to her pain experience. At a multidisciplinary meeting, the team decided that physiotherapy was needed and walking aids required. Repositioning and an alternating pressure mattress were initiated because of the pressure ulcers. A dietitian makes weekly visits to optimize her food condition.

3.3.2   Case 2: Older Patient with Chronic Pain Due to Cancer

Mr. Smith is a 67-year-old man. He was diagnosed with primary lung cancer 2 years ago and underwent surgery and chemotherapy. A few months ago, he began experiencing moderate pain. The oncologist decided to take a CT scan, which revealed metastases. After approximately 2 months on naproxen, Mr. Smith complained of increasing episodes of intense bone pain. The pain episodes have increased in frequency and severity during the last few weeks, and Mr. Smith has asked his GP for increased pain relief given the frequency and severity of these episodes. His problem with coughing up blood has also worsened recently, and he feels tired and weak. His loss of appetite is making his physical condition worse, and he has suffered from constipation since his dietary intake has reduced. Fortunately, the support of his family makes a huge difference in encouraging him not to give up with his treatment.

3.3.3   Case 3: Older Patient with Cognitive Impairment Due to Dementia

An 85-year-old woman, Mrs. Lander, has been brought to the physician by her son-in-law. He reports that lately she has been less active and increasingly withdraws from social activities. A year ago she was living fully independently and enjoyed things like baking and going out for a walk. Nowadays she is unable to prepare a meal by herself and she rarely leaves the house. Her physical condition is deteriorating. She has lost weight, about 5 kg in the past 6 months. She has no significant medical history and is relatively healthy given her age. When her daughter mentioned that she was worried about her, she became annoyed and resistant. Her daughter visits more frequently nowadays and is concerned that her mother stays in bed during the day and does not want to take a shower anymore. Assessment reveals no depressive symptoms but she has a mini-mental state examination (MMSE) score of 17/30, indicating mild to moderate cognitive impairment. This is in line with her verbal abilities, which have declined. Lately she has also become more forgetful and increasingly resistant to help and support, especially in the morning when the district nurse visits to assist her with ADLs. Getting out of bed seems to be more and more of a struggle. Miss Lander displays aggressive behavior and screams for help. Because of this behavior, during the consultation, the physician asks Mrs. Lander if she is in pain. Her response is unclear and she changes the topic to talk about other issues, so it seems that Miss Lander does not understand the question about pain. The physician is not convinced that Mrs. Lander is free of pain and asks the district nurse to monitor here pain when administering morning care.

3.4   Screening

We know that older adults suffer from pain (Osterbrink et al. 2012; Lukas et al. 2015; Häuser et al. 2014) and that screening helps to identify those who are in pain as early as possible (Lipschick et al. 2009). Pain is a symptom with high prevalence, and nurses have to deal with it in all healthcare settings—community and hospital based as well as in acute or chronic care situations.

Currently very little evidence is available regarding the positive outcomes of screening for pain in older adults and how this may relate to pain reduction, physical or psychological improvements, and improvement in the quality of life (German Pain Society and DZNE 2017). Nevertheless, it is expected that regular screening in the form of a question may reduce barriers and enhance pain therapy (Kaasalainen et al. 2012), and the screening approach will support an awareness of pain characteristics and the identification of risk factors for pain in older adults (Kompetenz-Centrum Geriatrie beim Medizinischen Dienst der Krankenversicherung Nord 2009). The high prevalence of pain in older adults makes this an important aspect of nursing in all healthcare settings, and screening for pain in older adults with variations in cognitive abilities poses particular challenges (Hadjistavropoulos et al. 2010). The following approach to screening will help to identify pain and develop a suitable pain management strategy, especially in older adults whose cognitive impairment means they are not able to communicate their pain verbally.

The guiding question in attempting to gain an insight into the current pain situation of an older adult should be straightforward, for example, "Are you in pain right now?" This question might be complemented by observations of typical pain behaviors (Hadjistavropoulos et al. 2010; BPS and BGS (British Pain Society and British Geriatrics Society) 2007; Herr et al. 2006). If a single question does not provide the information needed, a numerical rating score (e.g., "rate your pain from 0 to 10") could be used as an alternative. A score of 3/4 or higher is often seen as an onset pain score. The use of a visual analogue scale (VAS) is not recommended for older adults as they can find it difficult to use such a scale, as demonstrated by its poor success (Ferrell et al. 1995). It might also be helpful to use other words for pain and focus on the most current health situation, for example, by rewording the question as: "Does it hurt anywhere?"

Nurses should have a high degree of suspicion about the presence of pain. Pain might be indicated by a "yes" answer, meaning the older adult expresses that the pain is present or the nurse draws this conclusion after communicating with the older adult and observing their behavior. Several validated pain assessment tools with observational measures have been developed to ensure a systematic observation focused on pain behaviors/characteristics. Such observational tools are used for screening as well as for comprehensive assessment and monitoring of pain. To ensure these are used appropriately, nurses must be trained in the delivery and analysis of the observational tools as well as the interpretation of the results. However, little more than brief training in using the tools is usually needed.

Nurses, nursing assistants, and carers of older adults with cognitive impairment should be aware that knowledge of an individual's behavior and daily activities/habits is a prerequisite for effective pain screening (German Pain Society and DZNE 2017; AMDA (American Medical Directors Association) 2012). This is important, partly because pain might be presented as a change of individual behavior or daily habits and not demonstrated by typical pain behavior, such as facial expression, due to dementia. These changes can be manifested, for example, as restlessness or changes in eating behavior that are more easily recognized over longer observation periods. Not knowing the person well makes screening for pain, especially in cognitively impaired older adults, even more challenging on admission into an acute care setting. If nurses do not know the person and his/her pain-specific behavior, in this situation, proxy reports of pain-specific behavior from carers or significant others from the person's support network such as nurses from community care or neighbors are essential in screening and identifying pain (AGS (American Geriatrics Society Panel on Persistent Pain in Older Persons) 2002). This can help, for example, to construct an individualized pain passport for the person based on previous experiences that include individualized pain behavior.

In the first instance, to facilitate a pain self-report, it is important to give the patient time to answer questions and, for example, to provide acoustic aids to enable a self-report. The screening question or observation should focus on of the present encounter and may be occasion-related or carried out during regular care activity (Sloane et al. 2007). Pain screening should be focused on both being at rest and during movement (DNQP (Deutsches Netzwerk für Qualitätsentwicklung in der Pflege) 2015; DNQP (Deutsches Netzwerk für Qualitätssicherung in der Pflege) 2011). During morning care, for example, nurses can ask older people about their pain and observe them in both situations.

In long-term care, a screening for pain should be conducted within 24 h of admission. In hospital, screening should be conducted shortly after admission to help the interdisciplinary healthcare team to commence a comprehensive pain assessment and create an individualized care plan to prevent or minimize pain for the older person (RNAO (Registered Nurses Association of Ontario) 2013). In hospital, although changes in vital signs (heart rate, blood pressure) are not the sole source of information regarding the presence of pain, if abnormalities are observed, they should lead to a screening for or comprehensive assessment of pain (RNAO (Registered Nurses Association of Ontario) 2013).

The results of pain screening (positive and negative, including information about the preferred method, and the pain terms used by the older person, or any difficulties such as hearing or visual impairments) must be documented and communicated within the care team. This is especially important in relation to individualized pain characteristics of older adults with cognitive or communicative impairment. This information will provide a baseline for comparison in follow-up screening or assessment (RNAO (Registered Nurses Association of Ontario) 2013).

3.5   Focused Assessment of Pain

Pain assessment should be a multidisciplinary process. According to the biopsychosocial model, such an assessment encompasses all dimensions of pain and is intended to support a decision on the further course of treatment (German Pain Society and DZNE 2017). The aim of focused pain assessment is also to determine whether pain is caused by newly occurring diseases or by the exacerbation of chronic pain. It should also be considered whether a cause of pain can be identified and/or whether disease-related interventions could have an influence on the cause of chronic pain (German Pain Society and DZNE 2017; AGS (American Geriatrics Society Panel on Persistent Pain in Older Persons) 2002).

McCaffery's paradigm (McCaffery 1968), "Pain is whatever the experiencing person says it is, existing whenever he/she says it does" focuses on the self-report of pain which is regarded as the gold standard in pain assessment. Self-report of pain can be used, for example, to assess the intensity of pain, which mainly refers to the sensory-discriminatory pain dimension and is important for the detection of acute pain. However, it is of equal importance to also include affective-motivational and cognitive-evaluative dimensions of pain during focused pain assessment.

Everyone should specify his or her individual pain threshold and pain tolerance based on his or her own experience and individual conditions (McCaffery and Pasero 1999; Wright 2015). The pain threshold is the point at which a person experiencing a nociceptive stimulus that is increasing in intensity rates this stimulus as painful. Pain tolerance is the intensity a person is willing or able to tolerate before withdrawing from a painful stimulus or situation. It has been shown that pain tolerance differs from person to person, e.g., in relation to personal and cultural beliefs. Nurses must identify the personal threshold and tolerance for each patient since pain is a subjective experience, often based on previous individual experiences. Pain is experienced by each person individually and therefore is expressed individually (Hadjistavropoulos and Craig 2002). Every person has their own "individually acceptable pain tolerance" and their "individually marked pain signature" (DNQP (Deutsches Netzwerk für Qualitätsentwicklung in der Pflege) 2015).

If the ability to self-report pain is absent, a hierarchical sequence in the pain assessment process should be followed (Herr et al. 2006; McCaffery and Pasero 1999) (see Table 3.1). In particular, the hierarchy of pain detection should be taken into account when assessing acute pain where physiological factors could give indications of pain (German Pain Society and DZNE 2017).

In the example of Mrs. Thomas, it becomes clear that she is in severe pain. This can be determined by assessing pain on the numerical rating scale (NRS) or a verbal descriptor scale (VDS). The VDS has shown to be valid and reliable and is preferred for older persons with dementia (Herr 2011). Prior to that, however, Mrs. Thomas showed challenging behavior, which the healthcare team rated as uncooperative. A screening or initial pain assessment could have brought about faster clarification.

Table 3.1 Hierarchy of pain assessment approaches

1. Self-report of the patient using a self-assessment scale (e.g., verbal descriptor scale, numeric rating scale 0–10, verbal rating scale)
2. Testing for pathological health conditions that may cause pain
3. Observe behavior (e.g., facial expressions, crying), using observational pain assessment tools (e.g., PAINAID, PACSLAC)
4. Pain report of family/proxy members
5. Physiological changes such as blood pressure and pulse

Assessing different pain dimensions requires a broad view and a holistic approach. When assessing chronic pain, it is important to consider the patient's experience of activities of daily living, quality of life, and dealing with pain and to focus on the motivational dimension and behavior (Snow et al. 2004). The McGill Pain Questionnaire (Melzack 1975) can be used for a comprehensive pain assessment. The tool can be helpful in assessing pain in patients such as Mr. Smith, whose case is outlined above. In the detection of pain in patients with cancer, the focus is not only on pain intensity but on participation in and quality of life and patients' pain coping. Mr. Smith's focus of care is particularly on his fatigue, his weakness, and his lack of appetite.

As the cognitive-evaluative dimension of pain is important, healthcare staff must select the right pain assessment approach and draw the right conclusions from it. Therefore nurses need to be aware of the cognitive status of patients. This can be particularly important after surgery or during a stay in an intensive care unit, when delirium is common in older patients (Herr et al. 2006). In the presence of delirium, the ability to provide information can fluctuate greatly and changes within a very short period of time. In contrast to dementia, self-report can be re-established when the delirium has subsided (Hadjistavropoulos et al. 2010). It is, therefore, important to screen for the presence of delirium, using established instruments such as the 4AT and the Confusion Assessment Method (CAM) or CAM for intensive care unit (CAM-ICU) to inform the choice of a pain assessment approach.

Older adults such as Miss Lander, with mild to moderate dementia, are usually able to give a self-report. It remains important, however, to use the patient's own words, e.g., "ow" or "it hurts," or to take into account individual statements like "aching" or "moaning" (Hadjistavropoulos et al. 2010; AMDA (American Medical Directors Association) 2012); otherwise it is possible that such vocalizations will be misinterpreted, and pain will not be properly assessed. As in the case of Miss Lander, challenging behavior may be mistakenly not assessed as pain. In cases of severe dementia, self-report is sometimes impossible and has to be supplemented with observational assessment (German Pain Society and DZNE 2017; Hadjistavropoulos et al. 2007; Verenso 2011).

In the literature, different statements are made regarding the ability of people with dementia to report pain. It cannot be assumed that all patients suffering from moderate to severe dementia are able to provide an adequate self-report on the pain they experience (Verenso 2011; Basler et al. 2001). Patients with severe cognitive impairment (e.g., dementia, delirium) often have difficulty in expressing pain and using a self-report tool due to these cognitive and verbal limitations.

If a behavioral tool is needed to assess possible pain in persons, for example, with severe dementia, various tools exist. Nurses should consider the following (German Pain Society and DZNE 2017):

- A proxy-rating tool should be used to screen for pain in older people who cannot provide a self-report.
- When an older person is asked about pain, communication aids (e.g., glasses, hearing aids) must be used, and ample response time should be provided.

- During the provision of basic care, the person's pain behaviors should be observed, and/or they should be asked about pain.
- When caring for cognitively impaired older people, healthcare staff shall ask about the person's possible pain.

Proxy-rating tools for pain assessment must be valid and reliable; the following assessment tools are recommended based on their validity and reliability in various reviews (Verenso 2011; Zwakhalen et al. 2006; Lichtner et al. 2014):

- Abbey pain scale
- Behavior checklist
- CNPI, CPAT
- NOPPAIN
- MOBID
- PACSLAC
- PAINAD
- DOLOPLUS

The format of the different tools available differs enormously: Some of the tools are in categories (PAINAD), and others include very detailed behavioral pain cues (e.g., PACSLAC). Although the abovementioned instruments have proved to be valid and reliable, the choice of instrument also depends on contextual aspects and staff preferences. For example, PAINAD is used worldwide because the tool is rather short (includes five items) and is often used in an acute care setting to assess pain in persons with cognitive impairments. The Abbey pain scale is frequently used in Australia and the UK (it is incorporated as one of the preferred tools in the national guidelines), while it is rarely used in other countries.

An up-to-date database of the tools is available on the following website: http://prc.coh.org/pain_assessment.asp.

Without any doubt, these tools help nurses to assess and report on pain in older nonverbal patients. However, it must be acknowledged that these are all aids to assist and support the decision-making process and are not intended to replace the clinical decision-making of nursing staff. Interindividual variability between patients with dementia is well known and always needs to be taken into account. This implies that patients can have pain-specific behaviors that are not even present in generic pain tools. All behavioral pain tools contain a facial expression component that has been shown to be a strong indicator of the presence of pain. These facial responses seem to represent a universal pain response as these cues are also present in all other pain scales for other nonverbal populations (e.g., neonates).

More recently, pain tools were developed to assess specific pain conditions in a specific population. An example is a pain tool to observe pain behavior in cognitively impaired older persons with osteoarthritis (the Pain Behaviors for Osteoarthritis Instrument for Cognitively Impaired Elders (Tsai et al. 2008).

3.6   Pain Monitoring

Monitoring constitutes the integral third phase of the pain assessment cycle, after screening and a focused assessment have been completed. The patient's pain-related situation and symptoms are regularly and systematically reassessed as long as pain or pain-related problems persist. The objectives for pain monitoring are:

- To detect and assess intended and unintended effects of pain-related pharmacological and nonpharmacological interventions
- To evaluate whether individual pain management goals have been met
- To establish whether and how pain-related interventions should be modified

Pain reduction, improved functioning, improved mood, and improved sleep quality have been suggested as clinical endpoints that pain monitoring should focus on (AGS (American Geriatrics Society Panel on Persistent Pain in Older Persons) 2002).

Pain must be continuously monitored in all patients with known pain and pain-related problems and in patients who receive pharmacological or nonpharmacological pain therapy. Instruments and approaches used for focused assessment of pain should also be used for the reassessment of pain in order to make comparisons over time. However, it is neither necessary nor helpful to fully replicate lengthy assessments. On the contrary, pain monitoring needs to be concise and readily integrated into clinical routines while at the same time sensitive to changes in the patient's situation in order to be useful, acceptable for the patient, and manageable for clinical staff. However, research on this topic is scarce, so the following recommendations are predominantly based on expert opinion (German Pain Society and DZNE 2017).

In cognitively intact, verbal patient's pain intensity, based on the patient's self-report, is the key indicator for pain monitoring. The same self-report measure for pain intensity that was used for the focused assessment should also be used for monitoring. Pain intensity ratings should be collected regularly, in intervals adjusted to the patient's individual situation.

Mrs. Thomas, from our first case study, suffers from acute pain due to a fractured hip and pressure ulcers. She is in acute hospital care, and some of the treatments she receives, such as physiotherapy, are likely to increase her pain in certain situations. In such acute settings, where changes to the patient's situation, due to interventions, disease progress, or complications, are likely to occur frequently, pain needs to be closely monitored. Pain intensity at rest should at least be assessed in the morning, once during the day, and in the evening, usually by a nurse or a nursing assistant. Also, when Mrs. Thomas receives physiotherapy or other interventions, the clinical staff responsible should ask for the pain intensity she experiences in that situation, to make sure that mean levels do not exceed set limits. All staff need to stick with the same instruments, such as the numerical rating scale, which was introduced to Mrs. Thomas initially. In addition to charting the pain intensity, the pain situation should be subject to discussion during interdisciplinary team rounds and with the patient, and further detailed investigations into causes of newly developed increased pain or changes to the patient's therapy may result from those discussions.

Mr. Smith, from our second case study, is on a slow, palliative illness trajectory due to his cancer diagnosis. He is supported by his family in his own home with the major goal of maintaining his quality of life. It is likely that his health will slowly deteriorate over time, including increasing pain. Sudden episodes of severe or very severe pain also have to be expected in cancer patients. Such critical situations may indicate a need for further investigation of disease progression. Mr. Smith and his family will need to develop a way of maintaining good quality of life despite pain and other symptoms. This means that some chronic pain may have to be integrated into his daily life as complete pain suppression may have other unwanted effects, such as sedation. Pain monitoring, therefore, should not become a focus of daily life but rather a necessary routine that should receive "just enough" attention. Daily assessments may not be warranted if the pain situation is stable, and weekly assessments may be enough in the specific case of Mr. Smith. When his health situation changes, or when he indicates increasing pain or other symptoms, pain should be reassessed more often.

In addition to pain intensity, other indicators may be regularly monitored in patients with pain, depending on the individual patient's situation and goals. Those indicators may include, for example (German Pain Society and DZNE 2017):

- Direct pain-related indicators, such as pain quality, localization, duration, etc.
- Unintended effects of the pain therapy, such as constipation, sedation, etc.
- Adherence to the pain management plan
- Mood
- Physical, psychological, and social functioning
- Sleep
- Delirium
- Indicators for abuse of analgesics

It has also been suggested that in chronic pain, monitoring should rather focus on "positive" indicators, such as quality of life and desirable social interaction of functioning, than on "negative" indicators such as pain intensity.

In chronic pain, patients should be enabled and empowered to monitor pain independently to strengthen their self-management competencies and self-efficacy (Lovel et al. 2014). Providing targeted and tailored education about pain assessment methods, documentation, and resulting adjustments to their pain management, for example, by adjusting PRN medication or consulting a clinician, is essential. As pain and pain management always affect the patient's social relations, the patient's family may be given an active role in pain monitoring, if the patient agrees to family involvement.

Pain diaries may help to document how chronic pain and pain-related symptoms develop over time (Hadjistavropoulos et al. 2007). They may also help the clinician to evaluate longer periods of time between consultations. However, the effects of pain diaries on chronic pain and symptom outcomes have not been studied fully, even though they form an integral part of current clinical practice.

Traditional "paper and pencil" pain diaries are now complemented by mobile apps for pain assessment and documentation that can be obtained from the app stores of Apple and Google. However, these apps have rarely been scientifically developed and evaluated to meet the needs of users, especially older adults (Free et al. 2010). Initial studies indicate that apps adapted to the needs of older adults may improve health outcomes (Klasnja and Pratt 2012; McGeary et al. 2012).

The challenge in monitoring pain in patients like Ms. Lander from our third case study lies with her impaired verbal communication skills. Behaviors that are used to gauge pain in persons with cognitive impairment are not necessarily pain-specific. Therefore, when such behaviors are newly discovered during reassessment, a thorough investigation regarding their cause needs to be initiated. There is a real danger in patients with cognitive impairment that behaviors are falsely attributed to either dementia or an already known cause of pain, while the real cause may be completely different. Given the high prevalence in patients with pain, delirium should always be considered a cause of altered behaviors.

Patients with impaired cognition may also be unable to communicate new causes of pain or pain exacerbation due to disease progress. Clinical staff must therefore be vigilant regarding any changes in patients' situation that may cause pain and may easily go unnoticed in this population.

3.7   Implications for Practice, Practice Development, and Research

At present, different instruments are available for self-assessment and proxy assessment of pain. However, as an international survey on the use of pain assessment instruments in people with cognitive impairments has shown, they are not consistently used in clinical practice (Sirsch et al. 2015b), and it seems safe to assume that in general pain assessment is poorly implemented in clinical practice. A specific challenge is posed to nurses if the patient's self-report and the nurses' observation of patient's pain behaviors seem to be incongruent. Both objective (nurses' observation) and subjective (patient's self-report) sources of information have to be taken into account in determining the presence of pain. If possible, further information from proxies should also be included in this process. Additionally, when pain is suspected or possible, an analgesic (non)pharmacological trial should be initiated. Subsequent pain monitoring will help to determine whether pain was present. Communication about pain-specific findings within a "collegial dialog" in nursing teams or as an interdisciplinary case conference will enhance the understanding of pain, pain assessment, and pain management in all members of the healthcare team. Furthermore, it will facilitate the unique process of pain screening and necessary interventions, as well as the identification of an advanced/comprehensive pain assessment in older adults with and without cognitive or communicative impairment after positive screening.

Only limited research has focused on how to best implement and perform pain monitoring in patients outside the acute care setting. Therefore, the intervals in which pain is reassessed and the methods and instruments used for monitoring pain need to be based on the clinician's judgment of the individual patient's situation, needs, and preferences. Future research should take a longitudinal perspective on pain assessment throughout the patient's journey with pain over months and years in different settings.

Pain assessment is an ongoing process that must not stop once a focused assessment of a patient's pain situation has been completed. Continuous monitoring of intended and unintended effects of pharmacological and nonpharmacological interventions is an integral part of the pain assessment cycle. The choice of instruments and approaches needs to be based on the patient's situation and individual shared pain management goals. New assessment instruments have been developed. An attempt is being made to automatically capture mimic change through electronic face recognition for patients with cognitive impairment or sedated patients. Future technological advances should aim to improve the interconnectedness of apps for pain monitoring used by patients with information systems used by clinicians. Systems currently available are still in their infancy and do not adequately reflect patients' and clinicians' perspectives. Internet-based e-health systems for real-time communication (including video consultations) and remote monitoring are currently under development. Whether this automated recording of facial changes and information systems will fit into a comprehensive pain assessment in which all dimensions of pain should be recorded and whether these improve care is a question for further research.

References

AGS (American Geriatrics Society Panel on Persistent Pain in Older Persons). The management of persistent pain in older persons. J Am Geriatr Soc. 2002;50:205–24.

Alfaro-LeFevre R. Applying nursing process. The foundation for clinical reasoning. Philadelphia: Wolters Kluwer Health; 2014.

AMDA (American Medical Directors Association) Pain management in the long-term-care setting Clinical Practice Guideline. Columbia; 2012.

Basler H-D, Bloem R, Casser HR, Gerbershagen HU, Griessinger N, Hankemeier U, et al. Ein strukturiertes Schmerzinterview fur geriatrische Patienten. Schmerz. 2001;15(3):164–71.

BPS & BGS (British Pain Society and British Geriatrics Society). The assessment of pain in older people. 2007. https://www.britishpainsociety.org/static/uploads/resources/files/book_pain_older_people.pdf. Accessed 23 Mar 2017.

DNQP (Deutsches Netzwerk für Qualitätsentwicklung in der Pflege) [German Network of Quality Assurance in Nursing]. Expertenstandard Schmerzmanagement in der Pflege bei chronischen Schmerzen [National Standard of Pain Management in Nursing of Chronic Pain). Germany, Osnabrück; 2015. http://www.dnqp.de.

DNQP (Deutsches Netzwerk für Qualitätssicherung in der Pflege) [German Network of Quality Assurance in Nursing], Expertenstandard Schmerzmanagement in der Pflege bei akuten Schmerzen [National Standard of Pain Management in Nursing of Acute Pain). Germany, Osnabrück; 2011.

Ferrell BA, Ferrell BR, Rivera L. Pain in cognitively impaired nursing home patients. J Pain Symptom Manag. 1995;10:591.

Free C, Phillips G, Felix L, Galli L, Patel V, Edwards P. The effectiveness of M-health technologies for improving health and health services: a systematic review protocol. BMC Res Notes. 2010;3:250. https://doi.org/10.1186/1756-0500-3-250.

German Pain Society & DZNE (German Pain Society & Deutsches Zentrum für Neurodegenerative Erkrankungen e.V.). Schmerzassessment bei älteren Menschen in der vollstationären Altenhilfe. [Pain assessment in older adults in long-term-care facilities]. Working Group "Pain and Age". AWMF Leitlinie 145–001 2017. 2017

Hadjistavropoulos T, Craig KD. A theoretical framework for understanding self-report and observational measures of pain: a communications model. Behav Res Ther. 2002;40(5):551–70.

Hadjistavropoulos T, Herr K, Turk DC, Fine PG, Dworkin RH, Helme R, Jackson K, Parmelee PA, Rudy TE, Lynn Beattie B, Chibnall JT, Craig KD, Ferrell B, Ferrell B, Fillingim RB, Gagliese L, Gallagher R, Gibson SJ, Harrison EL, Katz B, Keefe FJ, Lieber SJ, Lussier D, Schmader KE, Tait RC, Weiner DK, Williams J. An interdisciplinary expert consensus statement on assessment of pain in older persons. Clin J Pain. 2007;23(SUPPL. 1):S1–43. https://doi.org/10.1097/AJP.0b013e31802be869.

Hadjistavropoulos T, Fitzgerald TD, Marchildon GP. Practice guidelines for assessing pain in older persons with dementia residing in long-term care facilities. Physiother Can. 2010;62: 104–13.

Häuser W, Schmutzer G, Henningsen P, Brähler E. Chronische Schmerzen, Schmerzkrankheit und Zufriedenheit der Betroffenen mit der Schmerzbehandlung in Deutschland. Schmerz. 2014;28:483–92.

Herr K. Pain assessment strategies in older patients. Pain Manag Nurs. 2011;12(3):S3–S13.

Herr K, Bjoro K, Steffensmeier J, et al. Acute pain management in older adults. Iowa City: University of Iowa Gerontological Nursing Interventions Research Center, Research Translastion and Dissemination Core; 2006. p. 113.

Kaasalainen SK, Brazil N, Akhtar-Danesh E, Coker J, Ploeg F, Donald R, Martin-Misener A, Dicenso A, Hadjistavropoulos T, Dolovich L, Papaioannou A. The evaluation of an interdisciplinary pain protocol in long term care. J Am Med Dir Assoc. 2012;13:e661–8.

Klasnja P, Pratt W. Healthcare in the pocket: mapping the space of mobile-phone health interventions. J Biomed Inform. 2012;45(1):184–98. https://doi.org/10.1016/j.jbi.2011.08.017.

Kompetenz-Centrum Geriatrie beim Medizinischen Dienst der Krankenversicherung Nord. INFO – Service/Assessmentinstrument in der Geriatrie. 2009. www.kc-geriatrie.de/assessment_1.htm. Accessed 22 Mar 2016.

Lichtner V, Dowding D, Esterhuizen P, Closs SJ, Long AF, Corbett A, et al. Pain assessment for people with dementia: a systematic review of systematic reviews of pain assessment tools. BMC Geriatr. 2014;14:138.

Lipschick G, Von Feldt J, Frame L, Akers S, Mangione S, Llewelyn H. American handbook of clinical diagnosis. Oxford: Oxford University Press; 2009.

Lovel M, Luckett T, Boyle F, Phillips J, Agar M, Davidson P. Patient education, coaching, and self-management for cancer pain. J Clin Oncol. 2014;32(16):1712–20. https://doi.org/10.1200/JCO.2013.52.4850.

Lukas A, Mayer B, Onder G, Bernabei R, Denkinger MD. Schmerztherapie in deutschen Pflegeeinrichtungen im europäischen Vergleich. Schmerz. 2015;29(4):411–21.

McCaffery M. Nursing practice theories related to cognition, bodily pain, and man-environment interactions. Los Angeles: University of California Students Store; 1968.

McCaffery M, Pasero C. Pain: clinical manual. St. Louis: C. V. Mosby; 1999.

McGeary DD, McGeary CA, Gatchel RJ. A comprehensive review of telehealth for pain management: where we are and the way ahead. Pain Pract. 2012;12(7):570–7.

Melzack R. The McGill pain questionnaire: major properties and scoring methods. Pain. 1975;1(3):277–99.

Melzack R, Wall P. The challenge of pain. London: Penguin Books; 1996.

Osterbrink J, Hufnagel M, Kutschar P, Mitterlehner B, Krüger C, Bauer ZW, et al. Die Schmerzsituation von Bewohnern in der stationären Altenhilfe [The pain situation of residents in long-term care]. Schmerz. 2012;26:27–35.

Reuschenbach B. Definition und Abgrenzung des Pflegeassessments. In: Reuschenbach B, Mahler C, editors. Pflegebezogene Assessmentinstrumente. Bern: Hans Huber; 2011. p. 27–46.

RNAO (Registered Nurses Association of Ontario). Assessment and management of pain. 2013. http://rnao.ca/bpg/guidelines/assessment-and-management-pain. Accessed 22 Nov 2017.

Sirsch E, Gnass I, Fischer T. "Diagnostik von Schmerzen im Alter: Perspektiven auf ein multidimensionales Phänomen" [Diagnostics of pain in old age: perspectives on a multidimensional phenomenon]. Schmerz. 2015a;29(4):339–48.

Sirsch E, Zwakhalen S, Gnass I. Schmerzassessment und Demenz – Deutschsprachige Ergebnisse eines europäischen Surveys. [Pain Assessment and Dementia, German results form an European survey]. Pflege und Gesellschaft. 2015b;4:316–32.

Sloane PD, et al. Provision of morning care to nursing home residents with dementia: opportunity for improvement? Am J Alzheimers Dis Other Demen. 2007;22(5):369–77.

Snow AL, O'Malley J, Cody KM, Kunik ME, Ashton CM, Beck C, et al. A conceptual model of pain assessment for noncommunicative persons with dementia. Gerontologist. 2004;44(6):807–17.

Tsai P, Beck C, Richards K, Phillips L, Roberson P, Evans J. The pain behaviors of osteoarthritis instrument for cognitively impaired elders (PBOICIE). Res Gerontol Nurs. 2008;1(2):116–22.

Turk D, Melzack R. The measurement of pain and the measurement of people experiencing pain. In: Turk D, Melzack R, editors. Handbook of pain assessment. New York: Guilford Press; 2011. p. 3–16.

Verenso (2011). Multidisciplinaire Richtlijn Pijn. Deel 1. Utrecht, Verenso.

Wilkinson. Reference missing from reference list. 2007.

Wilkinson J. Nursing process and critical thinking. Pearson: Upper Saddle River; 2012.

Williams A, Craig K. Updating the definition of pain. Pain. 2016;157(11):2420–3. https://doi.org/10.1097/j.pain.0000000000000613.

Wright S. Pain management in nursing practice. Los Angeles: Sage; 2015.

Zwakhalen SM, Hamers JP, Berger MP. The psychometric quality and clinical usefulness of three pain assessment tools for elderly people with dementia. Pain. 2006;126(1–3):210–20.

Non-pharmacological Management of Pain in the Elderly

4

Carol Mackintosh-Franklin

Abstract

Pain in the elderly is an increasing problem with increasing life expectancy resulting in many people living for longer with a range of age-related debilitating and painful conditions. Management of pain in the elderly can be complex due to increasing fragility, cognitive impairment and the presence of comorbidities and polypharmacy. Non-pharmacological methods of pain relief would appear to offer a solution to many of these problems. Overall the evidence for the effective use of many non-pharmacological therapies in pain management for the elderly is limited. Most effective measures appear to be those which support self-help, those which provide distraction and promote exercise and the use of superficial heat/cold. There is limited evidence to support the use of most complementary and alternative medicines (CAMs) including dietary supplements, and the role of psychological therapy is limited to improvements in mood states such as anxiety and depression. However due to the low incidence of adverse events, any non-pharmacological therapy which is perceived as offering some relief from suffering by the individual may have personal value.

4.1 Introduction

The extent of pain experienced by the elderly is difficult to estimate, although recent figures from the United States Institute of Medicine (2011) suggest over 116 million American adults suffer from persistent pain. In the United Kingdom (UK), The

C. Mackintosh-Franklin
Division of Nursing, Midwifery and Social Work, University of Manchester, Manchester, UK
e-mail: carolyn.mackintosh-franklin@manchester.ac.uk

© Springer International Publishing AG, part of Springer Nature 2018
G. Pickering et al. (eds.), *Pain Management in Older Adults*, Perspectives in Nursing Management and Care for Older Adults, https://doi.org/10.1007/978-3-319-71694-7_4

British Geriatric Society (2013) estimates the prevalence of current pain in the total elderly population as between 20 and 46%, with the incidence of chronic pain in the elderly living in the community between 25 and 76% increasing in the residential care home population to 83–93%. Although these figures should be treated with caution as they are subject to numerous methodological difficulties, it is clear that pain in the elderly is a huge problem and with the predicted global rise in the elderly population is unlikely to improve (Schofield 2016).

Causes of pain in the elderly are easier to establish due to the prevalence of age-related degenerative diseases, arthritis, osteoporosis and peripheral vascular disease (Takai et al. 2010), and fall into three common body areas: the back, leg/knee, hip and other joints.

The impact of poorly managed pain is also easier to identify, resulting in reduced quality of life, poor sleep and altered social activities (Brown et al. 2011) as well as slower cognitive function, increased psychological distress and a greater risk of developing a mood disorder such as anxiety and depression (Keefe et al. 2013). The difficulty of managing pain in the elderly is also compounded by age-related increases in comorbid medical conditions, polypharmacy and the increased risk of developing a form of cognitive impairment, specifically dementia (Bruckenthal et al. 2016).

This has led some authors to reject the current medical model that is so dominant in Western health care as unsuited to the treatment of persistent/chronic pain conditions, citing as evidence its failure to recognise the presence of pain without pathology, the ineffectiveness of many pharmacological interventions, their unwanted side effects and the need to take into account the multidimensional psychosocial factors which are integral to each individual's pain experience (Brown et al. 2011; Keefe et al. 2013).

This complex picture in part explains the difficulties of effectively managing pain in the elderly population. These failings in pain management have led many pain sufferers, carers and researchers to explore alternative approaches to obtaining effective relief. Tse et al. (2012) identified over 70% of residents in a sample of six residential care homes already used non-pharmacological measures to gain relief. Figures obtained by Bruckenthal et al. (2016) on use of alternative pain relief methods in the community similarly suggest 73% of people over 50 already using some form of complementary therapy specifically to reduce or treat a painful condition.

The recognition of the need to seek alternative non-pharmacological approaches to the management of pain in the elderly is clear and appears to be growing (Tobias et al. 2014), and this chapter aims to identify and explore some of the non-pharmacological approaches which may offer some relief to elderly pain sufferers.

4.2 Self-Management of Pain

Although many elderly people experiencing pain would like more attention paid to their pain by medical staff (Karttunen et al. 2014), most of the alternative or non-pharmacological pain interventions currently available require a degree of self-management. Information about self-management choices appears limited; Geilser and Cheung (2015) found most people using these approaches obtained very little information about them from health-care professionals and instead information was largely gained from family and friends; consequently education for self-management may play an important role in relieving pain in the elderly.

Reid et al. (2008) in an evidence review of 27 educational programmes concluded that they may be of benefit to older people with chronic pain, whilst more recently Platts-Mills et al. (2016) and Wilson et al. (2015) both reported on the effectiveness of educational self-management programmes for older people experiencing musculoskeletal pain, resulting in an increase in personal confidence to manage their own pain and reduction in pharmacological dependency. However The British Geriatric Society (2013) in a review of a range of self-management approaches concluded that the long-term effectiveness of these programmes was unclear and only those with longer-term support which are not delivered in isolation were likely to demonstrate improvements in pain relief and function.

Self-management may take many forms, but as an example, Porcheret et al. (2007) identified the two commonest self-management interventions recommended for the elderly with knee pain as exercise and weight loss, with self-care in these two areas as a more important aspect of knee pain management than medical or pharmacological interventions. This is supported in the most recent recommendations by the UK-based National Institute for Health and Care excellence (NICE) guidance (2014) on "Osteoarthritis: care and management" which advocates local muscle strengthening exercise as the core treatment for knee pain.

4.3 Distraction

Distraction as a means of minimising pain is based on the simple premise that a person has limited capacity to process information, and therefore by focusing attention on one thing, e.g. watching television or listening to music, they are able to pay less attention to other things such as pain. This distraction can be both external, so focusing on something outside of the person, and internal using some form of mental distraction such as guided imagery/relaxation (McCaffery and Pasero 1999).

Distraction can take many forms including individual self-developed activities which the person has found work for them; more formal distraction techniques such as relaxation, exercise and use of music; or more therapeutic therapies including specific psychological interventions to support the development of cognitive processes which move attention away from the person's pain.

It is important to note that many of the different non-pharmacological methods of relieving pain included in this chapter involve an element of distraction, including exercise, most complementary therapies and most psychological therapies. From available literature on these methods, it's currently unclear how much of the identified positive effect on pain relief is as a consequence of the intervention/therapy, or more simply as a distraction from the pain, and the role of distraction should always be considered when assessing the efficacy of most non-pharmacological pain interventions.

The efficacy of distraction as a means of reducing pain is variable across individuals and circumstances. Most studies focusing on distraction as the sole method of pain relief concentrate on turning attention away from episodes of brief procedural pain, and its value in the elderly and those with long-term and chronic pain is unclear. In chronic pain its usefulness has been closely linked to the individual pain sufferers' propensity to catastrophise their condition under the premise that people who are more prone to catastrophise their pain are likely to be paying more attention to it, and therefore the effect of distraction is more pronounced (Schreiber et al. 2014).

The use of music is one of the most commonly reported specific distraction methods with some evidence to support its use both for the reduction of pain and the management of anxiety and depression (Guetin et al. 2012; Bruckenthal et al. 2016; Quach and Lee 2017). Korban et al. (2014) used relaxing music to investigate its effect on people experiencing neuropathic pain. Thirty participants listened to 60 min of music via headphones. Pain scores at 30 and 60 min post-intervention showed a reduction in pain intensity which had a positive cumulative effect. It is generally considered to be low cost and with minimal adverse reactions, making music distraction suitable for use in most environments.

When considering non-pharmacological interventions for pain relief, distraction is a useful adjunct; however, it may have limited effect on people with cognitive impairment through an inability to focus their attention elsewhere. Additionally there is a danger that a person who can be distracted from their pain no longer looks like someone who is in pain, and this can lead to doubts about their pain from family, friends and carers. Furthermore it is possible that whilst distracted the person with pain may be more active than normal and this can lead to an increase in their pain symptoms once the distraction is removed (McCaffery and Pasero 1999).

4.4   Exercise and Increase in Physical Activity

The most commonly reported non-pharmacological self-management technique to relieve pain in the elderly is an increase in exercise and physical activity. Physical inactivity is common in the elderly population and can by itself lead to increased levels of disability and reduction in quality of life independent of any under lying medical conditions.

Two recent Cochrane reviews by Fransen et al. (2015) and Geneen et al. (2017) have both looked at the impact of physical activity on knee pain caused by osteoarthritis and chronic pain in general.

When focusing on knee pain, Fransen et al. (2015) identified 54 studies from which they were able to extract data, of which 44 were deemed high-quality trials. Findings for immediate post-treatment pain relief on a 100-point scale in the exercise groups indicated a reduction of 12 points, with physical function improved by 10 points and quality of life by 4 points on a similar 100-point scale. In the 12 studies which included 6-month follow-ups, these findings were sustained with a reduction in knee pain of 6 points and an improvement of 3 points on similar 100-point scales for physical function. The review concluded that the overall effectiveness of exercise on pain in the immediate post-treatment period was moderate, with a small longer-term sustained effect.

Although this moderate to small finding could be considered disappointing, importantly Fransen et al. note that this effect size is directly comparable with the use of non-steroidal anti-inflammatory drugs (NSAIDs) for the same condition, and given the low report of adverse effects of exercise as opposed to the many adverse effects associated with taking long-term NSAIDs (National Institute for Health and Care Excellence 2014), exercise should not be excluded as a minimally important clinical treatment.

Geneen et al. (2017) focused on systematic reviews of chronic pain and the effectiveness of different types of physical activity for reducing pain severity, improving quality of life, physical function and the acceptability to the health-care user. They identified 21 reviews covering 381 studies, across a range of specifically named painful conditions, e.g. osteoarthritis. Findings from the review suggested that individually delivered programmes have a greater effect than class- or home-based exercise programmes, with implications for planning of future exercise activities/programmes.

For pain severity 18 out of the 21 reviews reported improvements in the participant's experience, whilst 14 studies reported improved physical function, with mixed results for overall quality of life. From these findings Geneen et al. were able to conclude that although the quality of the studies was highly variable with some inconsistency in effects, the lack of adverse events meant on balance exercise was likely to have a positive effect on pain severity, physical function and quality of life.

Importantly Geneen et al. were able to identify that although exercise may result in short-term soreness due to undertaking increased physical activities, this rapidly subsided. Additionally exercise quickly became acceptable to the participants and was unlikely to cause any additional harm to people with chronic pain who may have been fearful of exercise exacerbating existing painful conditions.

Neither of these two Cochrane reviews looked specifically at the elderly population although it's likely that given the range of medical conditions included in these studies, many older people were involved. The lack of focus specifically on the elderly population is a common criticism (The British Geriatric Society 2013), and National Institute for Health and Care Excellence (2014) highlights the lack of data focusing on the very elderly calling for much more extensive research in this area to be undertaken.

Although findings from these two Cochrane reviews are useful at supporting the use of exercise as a non-pharmacological means of reducing pain. When considering the implementation of exercise in clinical practice, some practitioners may feel that more detail is required. Exercise regimes vary considerably and are led by a variety of practitioners, from physiotherapists to volunteers, and take place in a range of environments from community settings to exercise in the home, as well as group activities of varying sizes and one-to-one exercise programmes. Perhaps opportunistically Ambrose and Golightly (2015) suggest this lack of specificity could be positive, allowing for considerable freedom and flexibility when prescribing or providing active physical activity for those with chronic pain.

Those studies which do focus on the older population tend to be based on the elderly living in some form of residential care or specialist elderly community, as well as a specific form of exercise.

Patel et al. (2011) and Park et al. (2017) both focus on the use of yoga in elderly retirement community residents. There are many types of yoga; Patel et al. state their study used a 12-week beginner's class in Iyengar yoga, whilst Park et al. used an 8-week programme of chair yoga. Both studies found that participants in the programme reported many benefits, including decreased pain, although the long-term sustainability of these improvements could not be ascertained.

Similar studies have also been carried out using Tai Chi as the exercise modality either as class-based or one-to-one interventions (Brismee et al. 2007; Tsai et al. 2013; Tse et al. 2014). Again these studies all report positive improvements in pain reduction in the participants who undertook the Tai Chi classes, with minimal adverse effects.

Unfortunately most of these studies use small sample sizes and focus on specific populations and/or conditions which make it difficult to generalise from their findings. In an attempt to reach some conclusions about the efficacy of Tai Chi as a pain relief intervention, Hall et al. (2017) undertook a systematic review focusing on its effectiveness at relieving pain in musculoskeletal conditions. Overall they concluded that the poor quality of most of the 15 trials they reviewed made definitive conclusions difficult and there was very little evidence of long-term effects. They were however able to establish that Tai Chi was more effective in relieving pain in the groups which received this intervention than the no treatment or usual treatment groups, although whether this was as a direct result of the Tai Chi was unclear.

When considering exercise as a primary non-pharmacological intervention for pain management, it's clear that the evidence base is currently limited, although it is highly suggestive that exercise in some form can bring about short-term if not long-term improvements in participants' self-reported pain levels, as well as a range of other positive improvements in general quality of life. The range of exercise options appears extensive with no specific programme as yet having more benefit than another. The key components appear to be programmes that support increasing strength, whilst promoting flexibility and endurance, and programmes which improve balance can also reduce the risk of falls (The British Geriatric Society 2013).

Self-management, specifically personal motivation, is essential for any exercise programme to be effective, and subsequently this means it's important that the chosen form of exercise is tailored to the individual need, but also where possible to personal preference (The British Geriatric Society 2013).

4.5   Complementary Therapies

When considering non-pharmacological pain interventions, there is a common association with a range of complementary/alternative therapies. There is no common definition of what a complementary/alternative therapy is, but the US National Center for Complementary and Integrative Health (NCCIH) considers complementary therapies to be "When a non-mainstream practice is used together with conventional medicine" and alternative therapies, "When a non-mainstream practice is used instead of conventional medicine" (National Health Service 2016).

In the UK the House of Lords Select Committee (2000) on Complementary and Alternative Medicine (CAMs) divided CAMs into three groups. Group 1 is the most organised and professional bodies for which there is some research available to demonstrate their effectiveness; this includes osteopathy and acupuncture. Group 2 includes areas which have limited professional regulation although there is some evidence they may be complementary to conventional medicine, e.g. massage, meditation and counselling, and Group 3 includes areas which lack regulation and have no evidence base to support their use, e.g. crystal therapy, dowsing and kinesiology.

The use of CAMs is difficult to quantify. Bruckenthal et al. (2016) suggest that 31% of middle-aged and older adults have used complementary health approaches, with this rising to 43% in the 65–70 age group, whilst Yang et al. (2013) found around a third of patients with knee osteoarthritis used some form of CAMs for pain relief. The most common CAMs generally used appear to be herbs and dietary supplements; in Yang et al.'s study, this was glucosamine, followed by chiropractic, massage and yoga. For those people using CAMs specifically for pain relief, the most commonly reported were similar: yoga, massage, thermotherapy and activity pacing (Bruckenthal et al. 2016).

4.6 Massage

Massage is included within the House of Lords Group 2 classification due to the very diverse nature of what constitutes massage and the training for those who practice it. In most forms it generally involves the manual manipulation of muscle, connective tissue, tendons and ligaments with the aim of improving individual health/well-being (Cooil 2005; Bruckenthal et al. 2016). Massage is thought to provide pain relief through a combination of physiological reactions, the responses of the skin to touch and friction causing vasodilation and stimulation of the lymphatic system, the physical elongating and stretching of soft tissues and the analgesic effect caused by stimulating free nerve endings (Cooil 2005). Massage can also be considered an instinctive reaction to pain through the simple almost reflex response of rubbing a painful area in order to make it feel better.

The British Geriatric Society (2013) suggests that massage has demonstrable benefits for pain relief, advocating the use of slow-stroke massage and "tender touch" as improving both chronic pain, reducing anxiety and promoting sleep; however the evidence base remains uncertain. Bronfort et al. (2010) in an evidence-based review of manual therapies in the UK found little to support the use of massage in those with knee osteoarthritis or fibromyalgia, although there was some evidence to support its use in relieving pain in those with chronic low back and neck pain. A recent systematic review and meta-analysis of the effectiveness of soft tissue massage for shoulder pain found only poor-quality evidence indicating a limited effect (Van den Dolder et al. 2014), whilst Nelson and Churilla (2017) in a systematic review of massage therapy in arthritis were unable to do identify any pain-relieving effect.

It's unclear if the use of aromatherapy oils enhances the massage experience although many reported studies using massage appear to use some form of scented oil (Bruckenthal et al. 2016). Cino (2014) used aromatherapy and non-aromatherapy hand massage on a group of residential care adults, all of whom had some form of chronic pain. Reported findings indicated a positive decrease in pain scores for all those receiving the hand massage regardless of the use of aromatherapy oil. However a similar study by Nasiri et al. (2016) comparing lavender oil with almond oil and a non-massage group for people with osteoarthritis of the knee found only the group who had received the lavender oil massage experienced observable pain relief. However the effect was limited to the immediate period post-massage and 4 weeks after the intervention the effect was no longer significant.

General conclusions appear to be that soft tissue massage, as opposed to deep tissue massage, is safe to use in the elderly population and can have positive short-term effects on reducing pain although the evidence base is limited and lacks methodological rigour (McFeeters et al. 2014; Shengelia et al. 2013).

4.7   Herbal Remedies/Dietary Supplements

There are a large variety of herbal remedies available with claims to help alleviate pain, many of which can be considered as dietary supplements and hence excluded from the strict regulatory processes which control pharmacological preparations. The commonest non-medical over-the-counter preparations used for the management of pain tend to be either glucosamine or chondroitin. In spite of the long-standing acceptance of their use for pain relief usually in arthritic conditions, general research in their use is limited, their overall efficacy is unclear and there are a number of concerns with their regulatory status (Wirth et al. 2005; Bruyere and Altman 2016; Bruckenthal et al. 2016).

Glucosamine is thought to have an impact on proteoglycans which are a key component in cartilage although how this brings about pain reduction is unknown (Reid et al. 2012). Although initial research in the use of glucosamine appeared promising, in recent years where it is available on prescription, its use has declined as a consequence of the availability of newer independent trials and specific best practice guidance on the treatment of osteoarthritis which have all cast doubt on its efficacy (Galvin et al. 2013; National Institute for Health and Care Excellence 2014; Runhaar et al. 2017).

Chondroitin is commonly used in combination with glucosamine and is thought to act by providing joint lubrication to protect cartilage and improve compressive resistance. Again its exact method of action is difficult to determine, and more recent and robust clinical trials have cast doubt on its usefulness to effect meaningful pain relief (Reid et al. 2012).

There is however some evidence that suggests when both glucosamine and chondroitin are used in combination they may have a beneficial effect on pain relief

(Provenza et al. 2015). When two recent related trials used combined glucosamine and chondroitin compared with celecoxib (an NSAID), they reported this combination to have a similar if not slightly more beneficial effect on pain relief than the NSAID, with few adverse effects (Sawitzke et al. 2010; Hochberg et al. 2016).

Other ingested herbal preparations/dietary supplements are also available but it is out with the scope of this chapter to consider them all. Evidence for the efficacy of many of these preparations is poor and the mechanisms of action are unknown.

There are also a range of herbal preparations which can be used topically that also claim to have pain-relieving properties. Of these many are related to the use of aromatherapy massage and are considered in this chapter under the Sect. 4.6. Other topical methods of herbal application are less commonly reported although in a small study Chen et al. (2015) looked at the efficacy of a cocktail of Chinese herbs used as part of a therapeutic bath by people with knee osteoarthritis. Overall they concluded that in spite of the variance in use, herbal knee baths did provide pain relief with no reported adverse effects and could be a useful alternative treatment method.

Overall the evidence for herbal remedies/dietary supplements remains poor. Little data is available specifically on the elderly and most evidence is small scale and of poor quality, with the value of these interventions for pain relief failing to achieve more than the comparator placebo effect in many studies.

4.8   Acupuncture

Acupuncture fits within the House of Lords Group 1 classification as it has a long history of use, some professional regulation and a growing body of research-based evidence on its use. It can be described as a technique for balancing flows of energy or "chi" within the body that run through channels known as meridians. It involves the use of needles to stimulate nerves, muscles and connective tissues, and it is presumed that its pain-relieving properties are caused by this direct nerve stimulation which may result in raised levels of endorphin. However its actual physiological impact is unclear, and there are few studies which focus specifically on its use in the elderly population. As with other CAMs, there is also considerable variation in how it is actually practised (Ali 2005; The British Geriatric Society 2013; Bruckenthal et al. 2016).

In common with most CAMs, the evidence base for the use of acupuncture to relieve pain, particularly in the elderly, is limited with a range of poor-quality trials and contradictory findings. Schiller et al. (2016) compared two different types of acupuncture with a sham for patients with osteoarthrosis and reported significant reductions in pain for both acupuncture groups. Taylor et al. (2013) reported on a meta-analysis of the cost-effectiveness of acupuncture for low back pain and concluded when used as an adjunct to standard care it had a considerable cost-benefit, although this was not the case when acupuncture was used as a stand-alone treatment. However Hinman et al. (2014) in a trial of acupuncture for chronic knee pain concluded for patients over 50 it was of no benefit for pain relief over a sham intervention.

Overall it appears that acupuncture as a means of pain reduction is safe to use with minimal adverse effects but has limited research evidence to support its short- and long-term efficacy (Shengelia et al. 2013).

4.9 Relaxation

The use of specific relaxation methods has a long history which has moved from informal relaxation approaches to more formal relaxation techniques. Relaxation can be defined as a state of freedom from anxiety combined with relief of skeletal muscle tension. It's generally considered to be useful for the relief of pain as an adjunct to standard treatment and not as a stand-alone therapy and may be useful as a coping strategy when dealing with both acute and chronic pain states (McCaffery and Pasero 1999). It has strong crossovers with distraction (see above) and guided imagery (see below).

4.10 Guided Imagery

Guided imagery is a form of focused relaxation which uses imagined visualisations of pleasant imagery to distract attention away from current unpleasant or painful sensations and may be useful as a technique to augment an individual's coping resources (The British Geriatric Society 2013; Bruckenthal et al. 2016). As in common with most non-pharmacological pain management interventions, the evidence base for its efficacy in the elderly is limited.

However available studies do suggest it may be of benefit, with early work by Baird and Sands (2004) indicating that guided imagery linked to progressive muscle relaxation could result in a significant reduction in pain in those suffering from osteoarthritis, with similar findings indicated in a 2010 follow-up study (Baird et al. 2010). Giacobbi et al. (2015) undertook a systematic review which identified seven previous RCTs that has used guided imagery and progressive relaxation on a range of arthritic conditions; although there was a high range of variation in the techniques used and length of exposure to participants, all studies reported statistically significant improvements in a range of outcomes including pain, anxiety, depression and quality of life.

Given the minimal adverse effects of such an intervention, it's generally considered a safe and acceptable adjunctive intervention to support the non-pharmacological management of pain.

4.11 Transcutaneous Electrical Nerve Stimulation

Transcutaneous electrical nerve stimulation (TENS) has been studied extensively since it was first developed in the 1960s. It consists of the application of electrical stimulation to the skin through surface electrodes. The stimulation can be high or low frequency with high frequency also known as conventional TENS as it is most commonly used. It can be used in isolation or in combination with acupuncture where low-frequency TENS is mainly used. Additionally the frequency pulses can be continuous or in bursts. TENS units are small and portable and suitable for use in a variety of environments, and they are also cheap to purchase for use without medical supervision (Cooil 2005).

Pain relief is thought to be achieved by the stimulation of free nerve endings under the skin producing an analgesic effect in the gating mechanism of the spinal cord and through a subsequent increase in endogenous opiates in response to this stimulus (Cooil 2005).

In common with other CAMs, the evidence base for the use of TENS in general as well as specifically in the elderly is limited with some suggestion that age-related changes can reduce its use in this population (The British Geriatric Society 2013). Additionally recent reviews have cast doubt on its overall efficacy in any age group for the relief of pain. A 2009 Cochrane review (Rutjes et al. 2009) which included 18 trials of TENS for knee osteoarthritis concluded that there was no evidence to support the benefit of TENS for pain reduction over sham, regardless of the type of stimulation used. This is echoed in the 2009 NICE report on the treatment of low back pain which specifically advises against the use of TENS for this condition.

Interest in the use of TENS continues with Simon et al. (2015) conducting a study specifically comparing the effect of TENS on different age groups. They found responses to pain relief were similar across all ages although noted that TENS amplitude was higher in the older age groups than the younger in order to produce the same degree of relief, whilst the 2014 NICE report on osteoarthritis continues to recommend the use of TENS as a non-pharmacological pain management intervention.

4.12 Use of Temperature

The use of different temperature states to relieve pain is also known as cryotherapy or thermotherapy. The commonest types of heat therapies include the use of ice packs, and hot water bottles, now being replaced by thermal products such as micro-wavable bean bags, gel packs and temperature-controlled wraps. These collectively are known as superficial thermotherapy and can be considered helpful as an adjunct to conventional medical pain management. Method of effect is generally considered to be as a consequence of the physiological changes which occur when the body is exposed to change in temperature; this includes changes in metabolic rate, haemodynamic effects such as vasodilation/vasoconstriction and an analgesic effect caused by the superficial stimulation of free nerve endings in superficial (skin-based) temperature therapies (Cooil 2005).

Although research in this area is small scale, reported findings suggest that the use of superficial thermotherapy can produce a therapeutic level of pain relief. In a study using alternate day heat applications for osteoarthritic knee pain, Yildrum et al. (2010) reported significant improvements in pain and disability, which are supported by similar findings in the later work of Petrosfsky et al. (2016). Arankalle et al. (2016) in a small study using alternating hot and cold compresses for the treatment of heel pain also reported positive findings for both pain relief and foot function in the alternating compresses experimental group.

When considering the use of heat, a further emerging field is the development of deep heat therapy using microwave diathermy focused on specific areas of pain; evidence for its use is currently limited, but it has potential to provide an additional pain management adjunct (Bruckenthal et al. 2016).

The use of cold as a treatment in its own right is less commonly reported; however Giemza et al. (2014, 2015) report on two small trials using whole-body cryotherapy for the relief of lower back pain and identified significant pain relief and improved function in the experimental groups exposed to daily whole-body cryotherapy of a temperature of -100 °C for 1–3 min. This method claims to use the body's own physiological reaction to cold to stimulate clinical pain relief. This interest in whole-body cryotherapy has emerged from the field of sports medicine but as yet robust studies on its utility for pain relief in any age group are minimal.

When considering the use of temperature change, there is some evidence to suggest that both superficial cryotherapy and thermotherapy can be useful in reducing inflammation and oedema with consequent relief of pain and improvement in function. Superficial thermotherapy is generally considered to be a cheap and practical method to use with few adverse risks, suitable to a range of environments (Cooil 2005). Evidence for the efficacy of more complex thermotherapy methods although promising is currently limited.

4.13 Psychological Interventions

It has long been accepted that the individuals' experience of pain contains many elements, physiological, emotional, sociocultural and spiritual, and that the subjective experience of pain is moulded by a range of psychological factors. The pain experience is also closely linked to individual mood states such as anger, depression and anxiety commonly recognised as the biopsychosocial model (Dallob et al. 2005; Keefe et al. 2013; The British Geriatric Society 2013). This understanding underpins much of the current research into the impact of psychological interventions/therapies in the management of pain. These psychological interventions can take many forms, and this chapter will consider the two most commonly reported: mindfulness and cognitive behavioural therapy (CBT).

4.14 Mindfulness

Mindfulness can be defined as a form of meditation where the individual pays intentional awareness to the present moment in a non-judgemental moment-by-moment manner (Bruckenthal et al. 2016). Evidence of its effectiveness in the elderly population is limited; however Keefe et al. (2013), The British Geriatric Society (2013) and Bruckenthal et al. (2016) all suggest it may have some positive benefit on pain reduction/acceptance, stress reduction and improved function. Morone et al. (2008) in a qualitative study of 28 adults all over 65 years of age describe positive results including immediate improvements in well-being which were sustained beyond the period of meditation.

4.15 Cognitive Behavioural Therapy

Cognitive behavioural therapies (CBT) use a range of psychosocial techniques in an attempt to alter beliefs and attitudes, increase a person's perceptions of control over their situation and try to modify any dysfunctional thought patterns. When used for pain, CBT focuses on specific patterns of behaviour and how these may have altered by exposure to pain and stress. The emphasis in CBT therapy is in working with the individual to support modifications in behaviours and way of thinking which enable them to develop more resilient coping strategies or to live with their pain in a better way. Skills taught may include relaxation, activity pacing, problem solving, distraction and changing negative thought patterns (The British Geriatric Society 2013; Keefe et al. 2013; Ehde et al. 2014; Bruckenthal et al. 2016).

Evidence to support the use of CBT in the elderly is available, although studies use a variety of different CBT modalities in a number of different settings such as residential care homes, community settings and Internet-based programmes, which make direct comparison difficult. Overall conclusions seem to suggest that CBT can be effective in reducing pain as a small to medium effect (Keefe et al. 2013), however its more significant effects are a positive improvement in areas such as depression, anxiety and self-efficacy (Nash et al. 2013; The British Geriatric Society 2013; Ehde et al. 2014).

This finding is supported by National Institute for Health and Care excellence (2009) who recommends the use of CBT as a treatment for adults with physical ill health who also suffer from severe to mild depressive symptoms. However when CBT is used specifically as a pain management modality, current NICE guidance is less favourable, with no reference to CBT in the 2014 NICE guidance on osteoarthritis and the National Institute of Health Care Excellence (2016) guidance on the treatment and management of back pain with or without sciatica only recommending its use as an adjunct to other treatment modalities.

Consequently the impact of psychological therapies as an effective pain management intervention in the elderly is difficult to determine. Reporting of adverse side effects from psychological interventions appears limited, and there is some evidence to support their use on the wider biopsychosocial aspects of the individuals' pain experience, particularly anxiety and depression, but evidence of their effectiveness in decreasing the intensity of the actual pain experience is currently unclear.

Conclusion

This chapter has considered a range of non-pharmacological therapies which could be utilised to support the management of pain in the elderly. Those reviews include self-management programmes, distraction, exercise and complementary and psychological therapies.

Priorities when planning to use a non-pharmacological pain management intervention based on the available evidence are as follows:

1. Self-management—encouraging and supporting individual pain sufferers to take responsibility for and learn to manage their own pain through some form of education.
2. Exercise—in all forms providing they meet an individual's preference and work to build strength and flexibility.
3. Distraction—reducing or diverting an individual's attention away from their own painful experience. This could include guided imagery, relaxation or massage as a distraction technique.
4. Use of superficial temperature changes—either hot or cold.

However it's important to add that these non-pharmacological therapies should be used as an adjunctive and not a primary treatment for the management of pain.

Interventions of limited or no proven value for pain management include most CAMs with the exception of those which may promote distraction and relaxation and psychological therapies except where they may be useful as an adjunctive treatment when comorbidities of depression and anxiety are present.

There are current limitations in the evidence base:

- Research specifically on the elderly population in any non-pharmacological pain intervention is limited.
- Where research evidence is available, most of it is of moderate to poor quality with small-scale studies lacking both internal and external validity.
- Where systematic reviews and meta-analysis have been available, results are generally inconclusive.
- Where research is available, it focuses on a limited range of medical conditions, mainly osteoarthritis and musculoskeletal conditions.
- There is no specific evidence of non-pharmacological pain management practices being used in the elderly with cognitive impairment or dementia.
- There is a need for larger, high-quality trials across the full range of non-pharmacological therapies.

This does not mean that non-pharmacological therapies should be dismissed out of hand, simply that the evidence base for most of them is weak and narrowly focused. Without exception all of the non-pharmacological therapies report minimal adverse reactions which means they may still have some value as an adjunctive treatment to both the individual pain sufferer and the health-care practitioner involved in the management of pain. The key to successful non-pharmacological management of pain is its adjunctive use, meeting the individual pain sufferer's preference and their personal experience of the value of the chosen therapy to relieve their suffering.

References

Ali V. Self-treatment strategies. In: Banks C, Mackdrodt K, editors. Chronic pain management. London: Whurr; 2005.

Ambrose KR, Golightly YM. Physical exercise as non-pharmacological treatment of chronic pain: why and when. Best Pract Res Clin Rheumatol. 2015;29:120–30.

Arankalle K, Wardle J, Nair PMK. Alternate hot and cold application in the management of heel pain: a pilot study. Foot. 2016;29:25–8.

Baird CL, Sands L. A pilot study of the effectiveness of guided imagery with progressive muscle relaxation to reduce chronic pain and mobility difficulties of osteoarthritis. Pain Manag Nurs. 2004;5(3):97–104.

Baird CL, Murawski MM, Wu J. Efficacy of guided imagery with relaxation for osteoarthritis symptoms and medication intake. Pain Manag Nurs. 2010;11(1):56–65.

Brismee JM, Paige RL, Boatright JD, Hager JM, McCaleb JA, Quintela M, Feng D, Xu KT, Shen CL. Group and home-based tai chi in elderly subjects with knee osteoarthritis: a randomised controlled trial. Clin Rehabil. 2007;29:99–111.

Bronfort G, Haas M, Evans R, Leininger B, Triano J. Effectiveness of manual therapies: the UK evidence report. Chiropr Osteopat. 2010;18(3):22–33.

Brown ST, Kirkpatrick MK, Swanson MS, McKenzie IL. Pain experience of the elderly. Pain Manag Nurs. 2011;12(4):190–6.

Bruckenthal P, Mariono MA, Snelling L. Complementary and integrative therapies for persistent pain management in older adults. J Gerontol Nurs. 2016;42(12):40–8.

Bruyere O, Altman RD. Efficacy and safety of Glucosamine Sulfate in the real management of osteoarthritis; evidence from real life trials and surveys. Semin Arthritis Rheum. 2016;45(4): S12–7.

Chen B, Shan H, Chung M, Lin X, Zhang M, Pang J, Wang C. Chinese herbal bath therapy for the treatment of knee osteoarthritis: meta-analysis of randomised controlled trials. Evid Based Complement Alternat Med. 2015;2015:949172.

Cino K. Aromatherapy hand massage for older adults with chronic pain living in long-term care. J Holist Nurs. 2014;32(4):304–13.

Cooil J. Self-treatment strategies. In: Banks C, Mackdrodt K, editors. Chronic pain management. London: Whurr; 2005.

Dallob RA, Lopez-Chertuidi C, Rose T. Psychological Perspectives. In: Banks C, Mackdrodt K, editors. Chronic pain management. London: Whurr; 2005.

Ehde DM, Dillworth TM, Turner JA. Cognitive-behavioural therapy for individuals with chronic pain. Am Psychol. 2014;69(2):153–66.

Fransen M, McConnell S, harmer AR, Van der Esch M, Simic M, Bennell KL. Exercise for osteoarthritis of the knee. Cochrane Database Syst Rev. 2015;1:CD004376.

Galvin R, Cousins G, Boland F, Motterlini N, Bennett K, Fahey T. Prescribing patterns of glucosamine in an older population: a national cohort study. BMC Complement Altern Med. 2013;13:316–22.

Geilser CC, Cheung C. Complementary/alternative therapies use in older women with arthritis: information sources and factors influencing dialog with health care providers. Geriatr Nurs. 2015;16:15–20.

Geneen LJ, Moore RA, Clarke C, Martin D, Colvin LA, Smith BH. Physical activity and exercise for chronic pain in adults: an overview of Cochrane reviews. Cochrane Database Syst Rev. 2017;1:CD011279.

Giacobbi PR, STabler ME, Stewart J, Jaeschke AM, Siebert JL, Kelley GA. Guided imagery for arthritis and other rheumatic diseases: a systematic review of randomised controlled trials. Pain Manag Nurs. 2015;16(5):792–803.

Giemza C, Matczack-Giemza M, Ostrowska B, Biec E, Dolinski M. Effect of cryotherapy on the lumber spine in elderly men with back pain. Ageing Male. 2014;17(3):183–8.

Giemza C, Matczack-Giemza M, De Nardi M, Ostrowska B, Czech P. Effect of frequent WBC treatments on the back pain therapy in elderly men. Ageing Male. 2015;18(3):135–42.

Guetin S, et al. The effects of music intervention in the management of chronic pain. Clin J Pain. 2012;28(4):329–37.

Hall A, Cosey B, Richmond H, Thompson J, Ferreria M, Latimer J, Maher CG. Effectiveness of Tai Chi for chronic musculoskeletal pain conditions: updates systematic review and meta-analysis. Phys Ther. 2017;97(2):227–38.

Hinman RS, McCory P, Pirotta M, Reif I, et al. Acupuncture for chronic knee pain. A randomised clinical trial. J Am Med Assoc. 2014;312(13):1313–22.

Hochberg MC, et al. Combined chondroitin sulfate and glucosamine for painful knee osteoarthritis; a multicentre, randomised, double-blind, non-inferiority trail versus celecoxib. Ann Rheum Dis. 2016;75:37–44.

Institute of Medicine (US) committee on advancing pain research, care and education. Relieving pain in America: a blueprint for transforming prevent, care, education and research. Washington DC: National Academic Press; 2011.

Karttunen NM, Turunen J, Ahonen R, Hartikainen S. More attention to pain management in community dwelling older person with chronic musculoskeletal pain. Age Ageing. 2014;43: 845–50.

Keefe FJ, Porter L, Somers T, Shelby R, Wren AV. Psychosocial interventions for managing pain in older adults: outcomes and clinical implications. Br J Anaesth. 2013;111(1):89–94.

Korban EA, Uyar M, Eyigor C, Yont GH, Celik S, Khorshid L. The effects of music therapy on pain in patients with neuropathic pain. Pain Manag Nurs. 2014;15(1):306–24.

McCaffery M, Pasero C. Pain: clinical manual. St. Louis: Mosby; 1999.

McFeeters S, Pront L, Cuthbertson L, King L. Massage, a complementary therapy effectively promoting the health and well-being of older people in residential care settings; a review of the literature. Int J Older People Nursing. 2014;11:266–83.

Morone NE, Lynch CS, Greco CM, Tindle HA, Weiner DK. I felt like a new person. The effects of mindfulness meditation on older adults with chronic pain: qualitative narrative analysis of diary entries. J Pain. 2008;9(9):841–8.

Nash VR, Ponto J, Townsend C, Nelson P, Bretz MN. Cognitive behavioural therapy, self-efficacy, and depression in persons with chronic pain. Pain Manag Nurs. 2013;14(4):e236–43.

Nasiri A, Mahmodi MA, Nobakht Z. Effect of aromatherapy massage with lavender essential oil on pain patients with osteoarthritis of the knee: a randomised controlled clinical trial. Complement Ther Clin Pract. 2016;25:75–80.

National Health Service. Complementary and Alternative Medicine. 2016. https://www.nhs.uk/Livewell/complementary-alternative-medicine/Pages/complementary-alternative-medicines.aspx. Accessed Nov 2017.

National Institute for Health and Care Excellence. Low back pain. Early management of persistent non-specific low back pain. 2009. https://www.nice.org.uk/guidance/CG88. Accessed Nov 2017.

National Institute for Health and Care Excellence. Osteoarthritis: care and management. NICE. 2014. nice.org.uk/guidance/cg177.

National Institute of Health Care Excellence. Depression in adults with a chronic physical health problem: recognition and management. Clinical guideline CG91. 2009. https://www.nice.org.uk/guidance/cg91.

National Institute of Health Care Excellence. Low back pain and sciatica in over 16s: assessment and management. NICE guideline NG59. 2016. https://www.nice.org.uk/guidance/qs155/.

Nelson NL, Churilla JR. Massage therapy for pain and function in patients with arthritis. Am J Phys Med Rehabil. 2017;96(9):665–72.

Park J, McCaffrey R, Newman D, Liehr P, Ouslander JG. A pilot randomised controlled trial of the effects of chair yoga on pain and physical function among community dwelling older adults with lower extremity osteoarthritis. Am Geriatr Soc. 2017;65:592–7.

Patel NK, Akkihebbalu S, Espinoza SE, Chiodo LK. Perceptions of community-based yoga intervention for older adults. Act Adapt Ageing. 2011;35:151–63.

Petrosfsky JS, Laymon MS, Alshammari FS, Lee H. Use of low level of continuous heat as an adjunct to physical therapy improves knee pain recovery and the compliance for home exercise in patients with chronic knee pain: a randomised controlled trial. J Strength Cond Res. 2016;30(11):3107–15.

Platts-Mills TF, Hoover MV, Burgh ET, LaMantia MA, Davis S, Weaver MA, Zimmerman S. Development and validation of a brief interactive educational video to improve outpatient treatment of older adults acute musculoskeletal pain. J Am Geriatr Soc. 2016;64(4):880–1.

Porcheret M, Jordan K, Jinks C, Croft P. Primary care treatment of knee pain – a survey of older adults. Rheumatology. 2007;46:1694–700.

Provenza JR, Shinjo SK, Silva JM, Peron CRGS, Rocha FAC. Combined glucosamine and chondroitin sulfate, once or three times daily provides clinically relevant analgesia in knee osteoarthritis. Clin Rheumatol. 2015;34:1455–62.

Quach J, Lee JA. Do music therapies reduce depressive symptoms and improve QOL in older adults with chronic disease? Nursing. 2017;47(6):58–63.

Reid MC, Papaleontious M, Ong A, Breckman R, Wethington E, Pillemer K. Self-management strategies to reduce pain and improve function among older adults in community settings: a review of the evidence. Pain Med. 2008;9(4):409–24.

Reid CM, Shengelia R, Parker SJ. Pharmacologic management of osteoarthritis-related pain in older adults. Am J Nurs. 2012;31(2):109–14.

Runhaar J, et al. Subgroup analyses of the effectiveness of oral glucosamine for knee and hip osteoarthritis: a systematic review and individual patient data meta-analysis from the OA trial bank. Ann Rheum Dis. 2017;76:1862–9.

Rutjes AW, Nuesch E, Sterchi R, Kalichman L, Hendriks E, Osiri M. Transcutaneous electrical stimulation for osteoarthritis of the knee. Cochrane Database Syst Rev. 2009;7(4):CD002823.

Sawitzke AD, et al. Clinical efficacy and safety of glucosamine, chondroitin sulphate, their combination, celecoxib or placebo taken to treat osteoarthritis of the knee: 2 year results from GAIT. Ann Rheum Dis. 2010;69:1459–64.

Schiller J, Korallus C, Bethge M, Karst M, Schmalhofer ML, Gutenbrunner C, Fink MG. Effects of acupuncture on quality of life and pain in patients with osteoporosis – a randomised controlled trial. Arch Osteoporos. 2016;11(34):1–10.

Schofield P. Pain management in older adults. Med Older Adults. 2016;45(1):41–5.

Schreiber KL, et al. Distraction analgesia in chronic pain patients. Anaesthesiology. 2014;121(6):1292–301.

Shengelia R, Parker SJ, Ballin M, George T, Reid MC. Complementary therapies for osteoarthritis: are they effective? Pain Manag Nurs. 2013;14(4):274–88.

Simon CB, Riley JL, Fillingim RB, Bishop MD, George SZ. Age group comparisons of TENS response among individuals with chronic axial low back pain. J Pain. 2015;16(12):1268–79.

Takai Y, Yamamoto-Mitani N, Okamoto Y, Kyama K, Honda A. Literature review of pain prevalence among older residents of nursing homes. Pain Manag Nurs. 2010;11(4):209–23.

Taylor P, Pezzullo L, Grant SJ, Bensoussan A. Cost-effectiveness of acupuncture for chronic non-specific low back pain. Pain Pract. 2013;14(7):599–606.

The British Geriatric Society. Guidance on the management of pain in older people. Age Ageing. 2013;42:i1–57.

The House of Lord. Select Committee on Complementary and Alternative Therapies. 2000. https://publications.parliament.uk/pa/ld199900/ldselect/ldsctech/123/12302.htm. Accessed Nov 2017.

Tobias KE, Lama SD, Parker SJ, Henderson CR, Nickerson AJ, Carrington Reid M. Meeting the public health challenge of pain in later life: what role can senior centers play? Pain Manag Nurs. 2014;15(4):760–7.

Tsai PF, Chang JY, Beck C, Kuo YF, Keefe FJ. A pilot cluster randomised trial of a 20 week tai chi program in elders with cognitive impairment and osteoarthritic knee: effects on pain and other health outcomes. J Pain Symptom Manag. 2013;45(4):660–9.

Tse M, Leung R, Ho S. Pain and psychological well-being of older persons living in nursing homes: an exploratory study in planning patient centred interventions. J Adv Nurs. 2012;68(2):312–21.

Tse MMY, Tan SK, Wan VTC, Vong SKS. The effectiveness of physical exercise training in pain, mobility and psychological well-being of older persons living in nursing homes. Pain Manag Nurs. 2014;15(4):778–88.

Van den Dolder A, Ferreira PH, Refshauge KM. Effectiveness of soft tissue massage and exercise for the treatment of non-specific shoulder pain; a systematic review with meta-analysis. Br J Sports Med. 2014;48:1216–26.

Wilson M, Roll JM, Corbett C, Barbosa-Leiker C. Empowering patients with persistent pain using an internet based self-management program. Pain Manag Nurs. 2015;16(4):503–14.

Wirth JH, Hudgins JC, Paice JA. Use of herbal therapies to relieve pain: a review of efficacy and adverse effects. Pain Manag Nurs. 2005;6(4):145–67.

Yang S, Dube CE, Eaton CB, McAlindon TE, Lapan KL. Longitudinal use of complementary and alternative medicine among older adults with radiographic knee osteoarthritis. Clin Ther. 2013;35(11):1690–702.

Yildrum N, Ulusoy MF, Bodur H. The effect of heat application on pain, stiffness, physical function and quality of life in patients with knee osteoarthritis. J Clin Nurs. 2010;19:1113–20.

Pharmacological Treatment of Pain

Gisèle Pickering

Abstract

Age-related factors influence the pharmacology of drugs and their efficacy/safety ratio. Pain treatment recommendations underline a more tailored approach. However, pain treatment in older persons with cognitive disorders, communication problems, or dementia is complex. This chapter reviews the challenges of adequate pain management in older persons.

5.1 Introduction

The frequency of co-morbidities, polymedication, and drug-drug and drug-disease interactions impact drug treatment (Arnstein 2010). Treatment guidelines for pain management and analgesic prescriptions for older persons have been developed worldwide, but specific guidelines for vulnerable patients are still lacking (AGS 2009; ACR 2008, Pergolizzi et al. 2008; Zhang et al. 2005; BPS 2007; APS 2005; Parsons 2017). General recommendations support a more tailored approach based on the optimization of treatment, anticipation of potential medication-related problems (e.g., falls, hospitalization) (Fick et al. 2003), co-morbidities, and a multimodal therapeutic regimen. However, pain treatment in older persons with cognitive disorders, communication problems, or dementia represents a real challenge for a number of reasons: pain assessment is particularly difficult in this population;

G. Pickering
Department of Clinical Pharmacology,
University Regional Hospital, Clermont-Ferrand, France

Inserm CIC1405 and Neurodol 1107, Medical Faculty, University Clermont Auvergne, Clermont-Ferrand, France
e-mail: gisele.pickering@uca.fr

© Springer International Publishing AG, part of Springer Nature 2018
G. Pickering et al. (eds.), *Pain Management in Older Adults*, Perspectives in Nursing Management and Care for Older Adults, https://doi.org/10.1007/978-3-319-71694-7_5

titration of action and dosage finding are cumbersome; behavioral and psychological symptoms of dementia (BPSD) are easily confused with pain; psychotropic drugs are frequently prescribed; and medications, sometimes inappropriate, may have a cohort of side effects, including delirium.

5.2 Pharmacological Changes with Aging

Pharmacokinetic and pharmacodynamic changes are associated with aging. A few reports suggest even greater significant pharmacokinetic and pharmacodynamic alterations in frail compared to healthy elderly persons (Shi et al. 2008).

5.2.1 Pharmacokinetic Changes

Absorption may be influenced by several factors including co-morbidities, medications slowing gastro-intestinal transit, chronic constipation, chronic laxative use, gastro-esophageal reflux, and dysphagia (Shi et al. 2008; Tumer et al. 1992). Furthermore, with transdermal absorption, significant inter-individual variability is often observed (Hammerlein et al. 1998).

Consequences of age-related changes in distribution are significant. Aging is associated with decreased lean mass, increased fat mass, and decreased total water volume; distribution of medications in the body is consequently altered (Hammerlein et al. 1998; Kinirons and Crome 1997). The distribution volume of hydrophilic medications (like morphine) is decreased, which increases plasmatic concentrations and requires lower dosing. Inversely, the distribution volume of lipophilic medications (like fentanyl) is increased, and this decreases their plasmatic concentrations and increases their half-life, often resulting in an accumulation of drugs (Hammerlein et al. 1998). Advanced age is also often associated with decreased serum albumin (Paolisso et al. 1995); this is more frequent in the presence of chronic disease or malnutrition, and results in an increased free fraction of the medication. These changes are, however, only clinically significant for medications with a protein binding higher than 90%, a small distribution volume, and a narrow therapeutic index (Grandison and Boudinot 2000).

Drug metabolism, liver mass, and hepatic blood flow decrease with age, which impairs drug clearance for flow-limited (high-clearance) drugs, with some authors suggesting 20–60% impairment of the intrinsic metabolic drug clearance (Butler and Begg 2008). The activity of phase I enzymatic reactions seems to be reduced, whereas activity of phase II enzymatic reactions is usually not modified (Schmucker 2001). Renal elimination, renal mass, and tubular secretion decrease significantly with age, with a 30–50% decrease in glomerular filtration at 80 years old. This may result in the accumulation of renally-excreted medications. Renal function and creatinine clearance may be estimated with the Cockroft-Gault formula, taking into account age, weight, serum creatinine, and gender (Cockcroft and Gault 1976). In older malnourished patients with decreased muscle mass, this formula overestimates creatinine clearance.

5.2.2 Pharmacodynamic Changes

Age-related pharmacodynamic changes often result in increased sensitivity of older people to medications and, consequently, increased occurrence of adverse effects (AEs) (Nolan and O'Malley 1988). More specifically, increased sensitivity of cholinergic receptors makes older patients more sensitive to AEs from anticholinergic medications, including tricyclic antidepressants.

Decreased homeostasis can explain the delayed recovery of basal state following impairment of a physiological function in older patients, including development of acute renal failure or gastro-intestinal bleeding due to the administration of non-steroidal anti-inflammatory drugs (NSAIDs), or sedation associated with opioids.

5.3 Analgesics and Pain Treatment in Older Adults

Pain evaluation is particularly difficult in patients with dementia and this central point is largely discussed in other chapters (e.g., Chap. 3). Suspicion of pain in demented patients may be raised by behavioral changes like agitation and aggression, and assessment of the efficacy of an analgesic relies on a systematic re-evaluation of pain and on the reliability of the evaluation scale. While agitation and aggression may be symptoms of pain in non-communicative patients, they may also be symptoms of dementia (Husebo et al. 2011). These BPSD may orientate treatment towards psychopharmacological treatment rather than analgesics, increasing the risk of serious side-effects caused by neuroleptics. In older patients with poly-medication and age-related pharmacological changes, treatment of pain will bring an additional pharmacological burden and the choice of the analgesic should follow expert recommendations. The frequent polypharmacy in older patients leads to an increased risk of drug-drug interactions and related toxicity (Pickering 2004).

5.3.1 Acute and Chronic Pain

Analgesics used for pain in older patients are the same as in younger persons. *Acute and chronic pain* (as defined in Chap. 2) treatment relies on the classical stepladder, which involves: step 1 – paracetamol (acetaminophen) or NSAIDs; step 2 – weak opiates like codeine and tramadol; and step 3 – strong opiates. Neuropathic pain is often refractory to these drugs and requires co-analgesics with antidepressants or antiepileptics. *Paracetamol* is widely used in older patients because of the high prevalence of joint pathologies and osteoarthritis and is recommended as the first-line oral analgesic (AGS 2009). It is recommended to use a maximal daily dosage of 3 g in older persons. Adverse effects are rare, with hepatotoxicity being the main safety concern in the context of depleted glutathione stores associated with malnutrition, prolonged fasting, being underweight, poor nutritional status, alcoholism, age-related changes of antioxidant status, or dehydration (AGS 2009; Pujos-Guillot et al. 2012; Pickering et al. 2011).

NSAIDs and the cyclooxygenase-II selective inhibitors (Coxibs) have a proven efficacy but a well-defined toxicity profile (gastrointestinal, renal, and cardiovascular), and NSAIDs may only be considered rarely, and with extreme caution, in highly selected older patients who have failed other safer therapies (AGS 2009). Studies have demonstrated that there is a high prevalence of inappropriate NSAID and COX-2 inhibitor (Coxib) usage in the elderly population (Abraham et al. 2005; Van Leen et al. 2007; Visser et al. 2002). Inappropriate medication prescription (especially the type of drug rather than the dosage) is frequent in older patients, and patients taking NSAIDs should be reassessed on a regular basis to ensure ongoing benefits, absence of toxicity, and drug-drug or drug-disease interactions (AGS 2009). A systematic literature review has recently suggested that an increased risk for accidental falls is probable when older persons are exposed to NSAIDs (Hegeman et al. 2009). It is interesting to note that topical NSAIDs have an efficacy similar to oral NSAIDs, with a low incidence of adverse events (Baraf et al. 2011).

Opioid analgesics are recommended for the treatment of chronic pain of moderate to severe intensity with pain-related functional impairment or diminished quality of life (Pergolizzi et al. 2008). A review on the use of opioids in chronic pain in the elderly, with a focus on buprenorphine, fentanyl, hydromorphone, methadone, morphine, and oxycodone, stresses that older patients respond to opioid treatment as well as younger patients, but tolerability is often a limiting factor. It is not possible to recommend the use of a specific opioid (Pergolizzi et al. 2008) and the benefit-risk ratio of each opioid should be considered as well as co-morbidities and concomitant medications. The general rule applied in geriatrics but very strongly with opioids, is to start with the lowest dose possible and titrate according to the analgesic response and AEs. Over the last two decades, opioid prescription has exploded, leading to an opioid epidemic with adverse consequences (Manchikanti et al. 2012). In older persons opioids are prescribed for cancer pain treatment but also in non-cancer pain and osteoarthritis. Osteoarthritis is one of the most common diseases of old age and a leading cause of disability and of chronic pain worldwide. Benefits and harms of opioids in the elderly are largely reviewed in the literature and are associated with a much higher risk of fracture (Solomon et al. 2012; Solomon et al. 2010) than other treatments (Gloth III 2011; Lussier and Pickering 2010). Opioid equianalgesia tables are available if opioid switching is planned but they are numerous and a consensus has not been reached (Natusch 2012; Syrmis et al. 2014; Shaheen et al. 2009). Constipation, nausea, and somnolence are common side-effects and should be anticipated, especially in elderly persons, by appropriate medications.

5.3.2 Neuropathic Pain

Neuropathic pain is common in older persons and remains a difficult issue. It has been demonstrated that this neuropathic pain often occurs in older patients with dementia and is often hard to treat and uncontrollable for the patient. Assessment of neuropathic pain is not easy, especially in older persons with cognitive disorders.

First-line medications of neuropathic pain include tricyclic antidepressants, selective serotonin and norepinephrine reuptake inhibitors (duloxetine and venlafaxine), calcium channel α2-δ ligands (gabapentin and pregabalin), and topicals like lidocaine and capsaicine (Pickering et al. 2017). The American Geriatrics Society revised some of the previous AGS recommendations on pharmacological treatment of persistent pain in older adults and strongly recommends that tertiary tricyclic antidepressants should be avoided in older adults because of the risk of anticholinergic, cardiac, and cognitive AEs (Gloth III 2011). Antiepileptics also have a number of AEs including dizziness, somnolence, gait disturbance, and falls, and reduction in doses is recommended (Pickering 2014). The known AEs of the classic drugs used in neuropathic pain may preclude their use in the frail older person. Topical and non-invasive treatments may be useful alone or in combination with systemic treatments. In older patients suffering from post-herpetic neuralgia, the 5% lidocaine-medicated plaster allowed a reduction in the use of antidepressants and opioids (Pickering 2014; Pickering et al. 2014).

5.4 Pain Treatment and Behavioral or Psychological Symptoms

Antipsychotics, anticonvulsants, antidepressants, anxiolytics, cholinesterase inhibitors, and N-methyl-D-aspartate–receptor modulators are used for BPSD (Sink et al. 2005; Kverno et al. 2008; Schulze et al. 2013; Kamble et al. 2009). Psychotropic medication is common in dementia patients with a prevalence ranging between 17% and 78% (Kverno et al. 2008; Schulze et al. 2013; Parsons 2017). Typical antipsychotics (i.e., haloperidol, thioridazine, droperidol, promazine) have major AEs including dystonia, tardive dyskinesia, cognitive impairment, and cardiac arrhythmias. Haloperidol showed an improvement of aggression, but not of agitation (Lonergan et al. 2007), and despite its poor safety profile is still used today. Atypical antipsychotics were the second generation of antipsychotics developed in the 1990s (i.e., risperidone, olanzapine, aripiprazole, quetiapine) and have largely replaced the first-generation drugs because of their slightly better safety profile in tardive dyskinesia. However, the risk of delirium (Ballard and Corbett 2013) because of anticholinergic effects and increased mortality (because of oversedation, dehydration, and cardiac arrhythmias) have been highlighted in the literature. The confusion of pain and behavioral and psychological symptoms of dementia may lead to an erroneous prescription of psychopharmacological medication like neuroleptics. Delirium may occur in 60% of those hospitalized and in 45% of the cognitively impaired (Lonergan et al. 2007). It may result from drug effects, and deliriogenic drugs, including antipsychotics, should be avoided in elderly patients (Maclullich et al. 2013). The combination of being elderly and cognitively impaired leads to a high risk of delirium with the associated increased risk of prolonged hospital stay, complications, and poor outcomes (Lonergan et al. 2007).

Pharmacological treatment of pain in the older patient is challenging because of co-morbidities that necessitate multiple medications (older patients are reported to take between 5 and 10 drugs every day) with potential interactions (Lussier and Pickering 2010; Pickering 2012) and with the risk of inappropriate medication prescription in approximately one in five prescriptions (Opondo et al. 2012). The challenges surrounding prescribing analgesics for older people are further amplified in the presence of frailty and impaired cognition (McLachlan et al. 2011), which may impact on the pharmacokinetics and pharmacodynamics of analgesics in this population and further increase its heterogeneity. Adequate dosage finding of analgesics relies on an individualized approach of pain management. Frailty is also associated with pain (McLachlan et al. 2011), and demented patients often present neuropsychiatric symptoms, which confusingly may also be symptoms of pain.

Conclusion

Optimization of pain treatment relies on finding the right benefit-risk ratio of drugs. The most common side-effects of all analgesic medications are neuropsychological, especially in long-term care settings (Hartikainen et al. 2007). Evidence for AEs of opioids and some antipsychotics (antidepressants, neuroleptics, benzodiazepines, sedatives/hypnotics), for example fall occurrence, has been well documented (Hartikainen et al. 2007; Leipzig et al. 1999). Beside the red flags that also have to be considered in the treatment of elderly individuals with analgesics, further specific challenges are associated with the pharmacological pain treatment of frail patients and patients with severe cognitive impairment. Because of the difficulties in pain assessment, titration and dosage finding are very cumbersome. Patients taking more than one CNS drug or suffering psychiatric illness need specific nursing attention from healthcare professionals. Polymedication should be hierarchized in order to avoid AEs and drug-drug interactions that are very common in the elderly. While pharmacological pain treatment is the first line, non-pharmacological approaches should be developed and always be tried and combined for a synergistic therapeutic benefit.

References

Abraham NS, El-Serag HB, Johnson ML. National adherence to evidence-based guidelines for the prescription of nonsteroidal anti-inflammatory drugs. J Gastroenterol. 2005;129:1171–8.

ACR American College of Rheumatology Ad Hoc Group on Use of selective and non selective NSAI drugs. Recommendations for use: an American College of Rheumatology white paper. Arthritis Rheum. 2008;59:1058–73.

AGS American Geriatrics Society Panel on the Pharmacological Management of Persistent Pain in Older Persons. Pharmacological management of persistent pain in older persons. J Am Geriatr Soc. 2009;57:1331–46.

APS Australian Pain Society. Pain in residential aged care facilities management strategies; 2005.

Arnstein RN. Balancing analgesic efficacy with safety concerns in the older patient. Pain Manag Nurs. 2010;11:S11–22.

Ballard C, Corbett A. Agitation and aggression in people with Alzheimer's disease. Curr Opin Psychiatry. 2013;26(3):252–9.

Baraf HS, Gloth FM, Barthel HR, et al. Safety and efficacy of topical diclofenac sodium gel for knee osteoarthritis in elderly and younger patients: pooled data from three randomized, double-blind, parallel-group, placebo-controlled, multicenter trials. Drugs Aging. 2011;28:27–40.

British Pain Society. The assessment of pain in older people. Concise guidance to good practice. A series of evidence-based guidelines for clinical management. Number 8. National guidelines; 2007.

Butler JM, Begg EJ. Free drug metabolic clearance in elderly people. Clin Pharmacokinet. 2008;47:297–321.

Cockcroft DW, Gault MH. Prediction of creatinine clearance from serum creatinine. Nephron. 1976;16:31–41.

Fick DM, Cooper JW, Wade WE, et al. Updating the Beers criteria for potentially inappropriate medication use in older adults: results of a US consensus panel of experts. Arch Intern Med. 2003;163:2716–24.

Gloth FM III. Pharmacological management of persistent pain in older persons: focus on opioids and nonopioids. J Pain. 2011;1(Supp l):S14–20.

Grandison MK, Boudinot FD. Age-related changes in protein binding of drugs: implications for therapy. Clin Pharmacokin. 2000;38:271–90.

Hammerlein A, Derendorf H, Lowenthal DT. Pharmacokinetic and pharmacodynamic changes in the elderly: clinical implications. Clin Pharmacokin. 1998;35:49–64.

Hartikainen S, Lonnroos E, Louhivuori K. Medication as a risk factor for falls: critical systematic review. J Gerontol A Biol Sci Med Sci. 2007;62(10):1172–81.

Hegeman J, van den Bemt BJ, Duyses J, van Limbeek J. NSAIDs and the risk of accidental falls in the elderly: a systematic review. Drug Saf. 2009;32:489–98.

Husebo BS, Ballard C, Sandvik R, Nilsen OB, Aarsland D. Efficacy of treating pain to reduce behavioural disturbances in residents of nursing homes with dementia: cluster randomised clinical trial. BMJ. 2011;343:d4065.

Kamble P, Chen H, Sherer JT, Aparasu RR. Use of antipsychotics among elderly nursing home residents with dementia in the US: an analysis of National Survey Data. Drugs Aging. 2009;26(6):483–92.

Kinirons MT, Crome P. Clinical pharmacokinetics considerations in the elderly: an update. Clin Pharmacokin. 1997;33:302–12.

Kverno KS, Rabins PV, Blass DM, Hicks KL, Black BS. Prevalence and treatment of neuropsychiatric symptoms in advanced dementia. J Gerontol Nurs. 2008;34(12):8–15.

Leipzig RM, Cumming RG, Tinetti ME. Drugs and falls in older people: a systematic review and meta-analysis: I. Psychotropic drugs. J Am Geriatr Soc. 1999;47(1):30–9.

Lonergan E, Britton AM, Luxenberg J, Wyller T. Antipsychotics for delirium. Cochrane Database Syst Rev. 2007;18(2):CD005594.

Lussier D, Pickering G. Pharmacology considerations in older patients. In: Baulieu, et al., editors. Pharmacology of pain. Seattle: IASP Press; 2010. p. 547–67.

Maclullich AM, Anand A, Davis DH, Jackson T, Barugh AJ, Hall RJ, Ferguson KJ, Meagher DJ, Cunningham C. New horizons in the pathogenesis, assessment and management of delirium. Age Ageing. 2013;42(6):667–74.

Manchikanti L, Helm S, Fellows B, et al. Opioid epidemic in the United States. Pain Physician. 2012;15:ES9–ES38.

McLachlan AJ, Bath S, Naganathan V, et al. Clinical pharmacology of analgesic medicines in older people: impact of frailty and cognitive impairment. Br J Clin Pharmacol. 2011;71:351–64.

Natusch D. Equianalgesic doses of opioids – their use in clinical practice. Br J Pain. 2012;6(1):43–6.

Nolan L, O'Malley K. Prescribing for the elderly. Part I: sensitivity of the elderly to adverse drug reactions. J Am Geriatr Soc. 1988;32:142–9.

Opondo D, Eslami S, Visscher S, de Rooij SE, Verheij R, Korevaar JC, Abu-Hanna A. Inappropriateness of medication prescriptions to elderly patients in the primary care setting: a systematic review. PLoS One. 2012;7(8):e43617.

Paolisso G, Gambardella A, Balbi V, Ammendola S, D'Amore A, Varrichio M. Body composition, body fat distribution, and resting metabolic rate in healthy centenarians. Am J Clin Nutr. 1995;62:746–50.

Parsons C. Polypharmacy and inappropriate medication use in patients with dementia: an under-researched problem. Ther Adv Drug Saf. 2017;8(1):31–46.

Pergolizzi J, Boger RH, Budd K, et al. Opioids and the management of chronic severe pain in the elderly: consensus statement of an International Expert Panel with focus on the six clinically most often used World Health Organization Step III opioids (buprenorphine, fentanyl, hydromorphone, methadone, morphine, oxycodone). Pain Pract. 2008;8:287–313.

Pickering G. Frail elderly, nutritional status and drugs. Arch Gerontol Geriatr. 2004;38:174–80.

Pickering G. Analgesic use in the older person. Curr Opin Support Palliat Care. 2012;6:207–12.

Pickering G. Antiepileptics for post-herpetic neuralgia: current and future prospects. Drugs Aging. 2014;31(9):653–60.

Pickering G, Schneider E, Papet I, et al. Acetaminophen metabolism after major surgery: a bigger challenge with increasing age. Clin Pharmacol Ther. 2011;90:707–11.

Pickering G, Pereira B, Clère F, Sorel M, de Montgazon G, Navez M, Picard P, Roux D, Morel V, Salimani R, Adda M, Legout V, Dubray C. Cognitive function in older patients with postherpetic neuralgia. Pain Pract. 2014;14(1):E1–7.

Pickering G, Martin E, Tiberghien F, Delorme C, Mick G. Localized neuropathic pain: an expert consensus on local treatments. Drug Des Devel Ther. 2017;11:2709–18. https://doi.org/10.2147/DDDT.S142630.

Pujos-Guillot E, Pickering G, Lyan B, et al. Therapeutic paracetamol treatment in older persons induces dietary and metabolic modifications related to sulfur amino acids. Age (Dordr). 2012;34:181–93.

Schmucker DL. Liver function and phase I drug metabolism in the elderly: a paradox. Drugs Aging. 2001;18:837–51.

Schulze J, Glaeske G, van den Bussche H, Kaduszkiewicz H, Koller D, Wiese B, Hoffmann F. Prescribing of antipsychotic drugs in patients with dementia: a comparison with age-matched and sex-matched non-demented controls. Pharmacoepidemiol Drug Saf. 2013;22(12):1308–16.

Shaheen PE, Walsh D, Lasheen W, Davis MP, Lagman RL. Opioid equianalgesic tables: are they all equally dangerous? J Pain Symptom Manag. 2009;38(3):409–17.

Shi S, Mörike K, Klotz U. The clinical implications of aging for rational drug therapy. Eur J Clin Pharmacol. 2008;64:183–99.

Sink KM, Holden KF, Yaffe K. Pharmacological treatment of neuropsychiatric symptoms of dementia: a review of the evidence. JAMA. 2005;293(5):596–608.

Solomon DH, Rassen JA, Glynn RJ, et al. The comparative safety of opioids for nonmalignant pain in older adults. Arch Intern Med. 2010;170:1979–86.

Solomon DH, Rassen JA, Glynn RJ, et al. The comparative safety of analgesics in older adults with arthritis. Arch Intern Med. 2012;170:1968–78.

Syrmis W, Good P, Wootton J, Spurling G. Opioid conversion ratios used in palliative care: is there an Australian consensus? Intern Med J. 2014;44(5):483–9.

Tumer N, Scarpace PJ, Lowenthal DT. Geriatric pharmacology: basic and clinical considerations. Annu Rev Pharmacol Toxicol. 1992;32:271–302.

Van Leen MWF, Van Der Eijk I, Schols JMGA. Prevention of NSAID gastropathy in elderly patients. An observational study in general practice and nursing homes. Age Ageing. 2007;36:414–8.

Visser LE, Graatsma HH, Tricker BHC. Contraindicated NSAIDs are frequently prescribed to elderly patients with peptic ulcer disease. Br J Clin Pharmacol. 2002;53:183–8.

Zhang W, Doherty M, Arden N, EULAR Standing Committee for International Clinical Studies Including Therapeutics (ESCISIT). EULAR evidence based recommendations for the management of hip osteoarthritis: report of a task force of the EULAR Standing Committee for International Clinical Studies Including Therapeutics (ESCISIT). Ann Rheum Dis. 2005;64:669–81.

Pain in Older Adults with Intellectual Disabilities

6

Nanda Cécile de Knegt

Abstract

People with intellectual disabilities (ID) have both intellectual and adaptive deficits resulting from genetic or medical disorders. Although scientific and clinical awareness has emerged that atypical pain responses in ID do not necessarily reflect pain insensitivity or indifference, pain assessment is still hampered by the risk of incorrect interpretations. Older adults with ID form a complex subgroup, because challenges in pain management from general older adult care and care for people with ID are combined. An increasing life expectancy demands an expertise in palliative care for the ID population, with its central concepts of pain treatment, quality of life, and communication difficulties. Although some categories of behavior appear sensitive for pain in adults with ID and pain diagnostic instruments have been developed, an individual approach is needed due to the many factors that influence pain in the ID population. This includes a tailor-made pain management plan with pharmacological and non-pharmacological interventions targeted at the pain characteristics of the specific individual in context of medical and psycho-social co-morbidities.

6.1   Introduction to Pain in Intellectual Disabilities

Various causes of cognitive impairment in adults (i.e., neurodegenerative, vascular, traumatic, toxic, anoxic, and infectious conditions) can challenge pain assessment and treatment, such as in the ability to report pain and ask for analgesics (Buffum et al. 2007). In earlier pain research, more attention had been paid to the subgroup

N. C. de Knegt
Department of Clinical Neuropsychology, VU University, Amsterdam, The Netherlands
e-mail: n.c.de.knegt@vu.nl

© Springer International Publishing AG, part of Springer Nature 2018   73
G. Pickering et al. (eds.), *Pain Management in Older Adults*, Perspectives in Nursing
Management and Care for Older Adults, https://doi.org/10.1007/978-3-319-71694-7_6

of intellectual disabilities (ID). According to the *Diagnostic and Statistical Manual of Mental Disorders, Fifth Edition* (DSM-5), ID is a disorder with onset during the developmental period that includes both intellectual deficits (i.e., IQ 65–75 or below) and adaptive deficits (i.e., personal dependence and/or social irresponsibility in activities of daily life) in conceptual, social, and practical domains (American Psychiatric Association 2013). ID are associated with genetic (e.g., trisomy 21) or medical (e.g., epilepsy) conditions and the severity should be defined on the basis of adaptive functioning (i.e., the level of required support) (American Psychiatric Association 2013).

Research on pain in the ID population has developed rapidly over time, causing a major shift in the conceptual and clinical approach of this topic (Symons et al. 2008). A persistent assumption about insensitivity (i.e., reduced sensory experience) or indifference (i.e., reduced emotional response) to pain has been used to explain case reports of atypical response in potentially painful situations (e.g., Devarakonda et al. 2009) and caregivers' descriptions of pain behavior (Biersdorff 1994). A steadily growing body of research findings has questioned the previously held view that an impaired pain expression reflects an impaired pain experience (Oberlander and Symons 2006; Symons et al. 2008).

Current pain researchers adopt the more likely explanation that people with ID have delayed pain processing or expression and atypical pain behavior due to cognitive and/or motor limitations in effective communication of pain (Oberlander and Symons 2006). In addition, technical innovations in DNA analysis, neuroimaging, and quantitative sensory testing has improved knowledge about genetic causes of ID as well as neurological and somatosensory functioning in these genetic syndromes (Defrin et al. 2004; Downs et al. 2010; Ferri et al. 1994; Miller et al. 1996; Priano et al. 2009; Price et al. 2007), leading to preliminary hypotheses about pain experience (e.g., De Knegt and Scherder 2011). Nonetheless, pain management of people with ID is still hampered by caregivers' general assumption of a high pain threshold (Beacroft and Dodd 2010) and tendency to under- or overestimate pain (Breau et al. 2003). This is alarming because caregivers of people with ID play a crucial role in pain assessment (Findlay et al. 2015), as illustrated by 47% of the healthcare professionals relying on caregivers' pain reports (Walsh et al. 2011).

Due to the clinical relevance of appropriate pain management for quality of life, the current chapter discusses the various aspects of pain in ID, targeting older adults.

6.2　Introduction to Pain in Older Adults with Intellectual Disabilities

The life expectancy of the ID population has increased over the last decades (Patja et al. 2000) to an average of 60.5 years in the USA (Lauer and McCallion 2015), depending on factors such as genetic etiology (Coppus 2013) and level of ID (Bittles et al. 2002). The aging-related risk for painful physical conditions such as musculoskeletal disorders is increased in people with ID due to a congenital vulnerability (Evenhuis et al. 2001; De Knegt and Scherder 2011). Medical conditions are highly prevalent (van Schrojenstein Lantman-De Valk et al. 2000) and include for example gastro-esophageal reflux disease (Böhmer et al. 2000) and oral diseases (Hennequin et al. 1999). As a result, the ID population is also often exposed to painful or dis-comforting procedures, such as surgery (Krigger 2006) and transfer from wheel-chair to bed (Van der Putten and Vlaskamp 2011). Chronic pain occurs in 13–15% of adults with ID (McGuire et al. 2010; Walsh et al. 2011) and negatively influences quality of life (Walsh et al. 2011). However, aging may further impair the ability to comprehend and communicate pain experience, due to cognitive decline and demen-tia (Herr et al. 2011). Taking the abovementioned cascade into account, the rele-vance of addressing pain in older adults with ID has never been higher.

6.3   Challenges of Pain in Older Adults with Intellectual Disabilities

Older adults with ID are confronted by challenges in pain management that are known from the general older adult care and from the care of people with ID (see Fig. 6.1). Challenges in general older adult care are described in the current book and include multiple chronic conditions, polypharmacy, slower metabolism of anal-gesics, and cognitive impairment (Reid et al. 2011). Similar challenges arise in

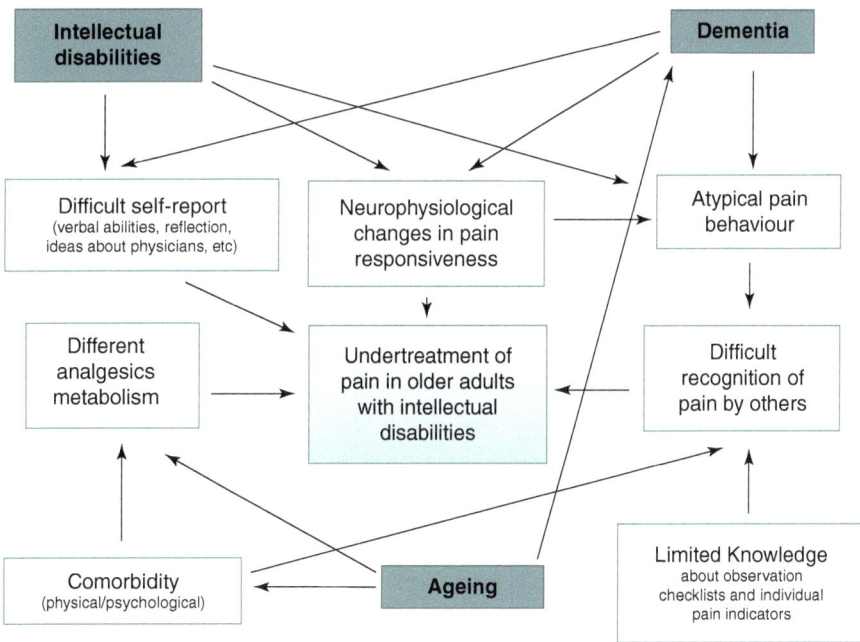

Fig. 6.1 Possible factors contributing to undertreatment of pain in older adults with intellectual disabilities. Inspired by Oberlander and Symons (2006)

people with ID (Oberlander and Symons 2006) such as multiple chronic conditions (Hermans and Evenhuis 2014), but additional challenges play a role. Congenital physical abnormalities originate from genetic syndromes, resulting in for example specific musculoskeletal conditions (De Knegt and Scherder 2011), or from a lesion of the central nervous system, resulting in for example cerebral palsy with spasticity (Schwartz et al. 1999). The general problem of pain diagnostics with the cognitive and communicative difficulties in people with ID is further hampered by atypical pain responses during pain and typical pain responses without pain (Defrin et al. 2006). The pain responses depend on the level of ID, learned behavior, and coping style related to mental age (De Knegt et al. 2013). A high pain threshold has been observed (Sinnema et al. 2013) and demonstrated (Priano et al. 2009) in this population, resulting in injuries (Sinnema et al. 2013) and possibly even death (Jancar and Speller 1994). The threshold may appear increased due to a delayed pain response (Defrin et al. 2004). Whether people with ID actually have a different pain experience is still a matter of debate, with some experts emphasizing neurophysiological abnormalities (De Knegt and Scherder 2011; McGuire and Defrin 2015) and others emphasizing our inability to recognize pain expression (Beacroft and Dodd 2010; Kerr et al. 2006).

Little has been written about pain management specifically in older adults with ID. Four literature reviews indicate the complexity of this topic, especially when dementia or palliative care is involved (Canning et al. 2012; Courtenay et al. 2010; McCallion and McCarron 2004). Staff in general health care settings such as hospitals would benefit from education about pain assessment in people with ID to better answer needs and to prevent 'diagnostic overshadowing' (i.e., incorrectly attributing a symptom of physical or mental illness to the person's ID (Ali and Hassiotis 2008)) (Canning et al. 2012). Such diagnostic error also occurs when wakening at night due to pain in older adults with ID is attributed to their comorbid dementia, leaving pain undertreated (Courtenay et al. 2010). Staff in specific care settings for people with ID need knowledge about aging and dementia in this population (Canning et al. 2012) to improve the recognition, assessment, and treatment of pain (Courtenay et al. 2010; McCallion and McCarron 2004). In the presence of terminal disease or advanced dementia, collaboration should be sought with palliative care centers in the general population for expertise about providing comfort for people with cognitive impairment (Canning et al. 2012). However, the challenge of communication difficulties in people with ID may necessitate a specific approach, such as a concrete reference to time and asking open questions (Tuffrey-Wijne and McEnhill 2008).

6.4   Pain Behaviors in Older Adults with Intellectual Disabilities

Pain behavior is an important chain in pain diagnostics of people with ID (De Knegt et al. 2013). This importance strengthens with age for three reasons: (1) increasing risk for painful conditions (Hermans and Evenhuis 2014), (2) decreasing cognitive and communicative abilities (Sheehan et al. 2014), and (3) possible decrease in pain tolerance threshold as well as inhibitory capacity (Paladini et al. 2015). Although caregivers use various behaviors to recognize pain in people with ID (Zwakhalen et al. 2004), a specific combination of vocal reaction, emotional reaction, facial expression, body language, protective reaction, and physiological reaction is sensitive for pain in adults with a broad range of age and levels of ID (Lotan et al. 2010). Still, individual differences occur (De Knegt et al. 2013) and atypical pain responses such as self-injurious behavior could result in caregiver misconceptions of 'challenging behavior' and high pain thresholds (Beacroft and Dodd 2010).

6.5   Pain Assessment Tools in Older Adults with Intellectual Disabilities

6.5.1   Standardized Pain Assessment

The advantage of standardized pain assessment is the use of psychometrically sound instruments to quantify pain, with which scores can be used for clinical decisions. As described in Chap. 3 of the current book, observation checklists for pain behavior and scales for self-reporting pain have been specifically developed for elderly people in the general population. Because these instruments are not (yet) validated for the population with ID, generalization of psychometric properties cannot be assumed. Until further research has been performed, clinicians should be aware that by using the instruments, pain behaviors could be missed and self-report of pain could be misinterpreted. Observation checklists (e.g., Non-Communicating Adult Pain Checklist) (Lotan et al. 2009) and scales for self-reporting pain (e.g., Pyramid Pain Scale) (McGuire and Defrin 2015) have also been specifically developed for people with ID. Due to factors such as cognitive and physical aging, dementia, polypharmacy, and co-morbidity, pain behavior and self-report abilities could change with age. By using the instruments frequently from adulthood, these changes may be registered in time.

6.5.2   Individualized Pain Assessment

Even standardized instruments that are well-validated for older adults with ID require an individual approach. Many experts advocate the need for such an approach in pain management for the highly heterogeneous population of people with ID (Doody and Bailey 2017a; Solodiuk et al. 2010; Weissman-Fogel et al. 2015). Pain observations and ratings should be considered for each specific person in context of the (pain) history, medical and psychological characteristics, and social situational factors. Especially for healthcare professionals in care centers, we recommend creating individual pain profiles in cooperation with clients, caregivers, and family members. Such a profile is a sketch of all pain-related characteristics, including reactions in potentially painful situations, possible pain treatments, and comprehension of self-reporting scales. Being aware of combined expressions that seem most sensitive for pain in a specific person is crucial for early detection and initiating pain diagnostics. Family and caregivers play a key role in advice about effective communication (Tuffrey-Wijne and McEnhill 2008). The individual pain profile is a 'living document': closely related to the Support Plan, embedded in the Electronic Client File, and actively updated with changes over time.

6.6   Pain Treatment in Older Adults with Intellectual Disabilities

Despite the heterogeneity of the ID population and its relatively young research field of pain, some excellent overviews about pain treatment in this population have been published and are used for the current section (Doody and Bailey 2017b; Oberlander and Symons 2006). After pain is detected in a comprehensive assessment by observing pain behavior and/or using pain assessment tools, medical examination is needed to diagnose and treat the cause of the pain. If the cause of the potential pain cannot be found on medical examination, then it is recommended to treat the symptoms and observe the effect of the treatment on behavior over days by also checking whether the symptoms recur after treatment ends.

In the complex population of people with ID in particular, it is vital to precede treatment with a well-documented pain management plan, in which family and the person with ID are involved and co-morbid medical as well as psycho-social conditions are taken into account from a 'total concept of pain' (i.e., physical, psychological, social, and spiritual factors influencing pain experience). As described earlier in this chapter, aging introduces the need to broaden pain treatment in adults with ID to the adjacent area of palliative care, with topics such as cancer pain and dementia. A pain management plan includes both pharmacological and non-pharmacological interventions that are evaluated for effectiveness separately. Due to polypharmacy resulting from co-morbidities, people with ID are at risk for analgesic failure in which analgesics interact with other medications (e.g., for epilepsy, gastro-intestinal reflux disease, infection, or challenging behavior). Analgesic failure could arise by: (1) incorrect selection of analgesic or dosage for type of pain, (2) genetic factors involved in an ability to metabolize medication, (3) the use of several medications competing for the same pharmacological pathways, and (4) neurological abnormalities underlying the ID. Neuropathy or inflammatory mechanisms may reinforce the pain. It is recommended to choose the analgesic based on the type and severity of the pain, the simultaneous use of several medications, and the choice between desirable outcomes (e.g., medication against spasm reduces pain, but may also reduce muscle strength).

During the acute pain of medical procedures, it is recommended in people with ID to use local anesthetics combined with sedation for anxiety, or to use analgesics combined with non-pharmacological pain relief. For chronic pain, the analgesic pain ladder of the World Health Organization (WHO) can be used to administer analgesics on a regular time schedule, complemented if needed with anti-epileptics, tricyclic antidepressants, or local capsaicin. Non-pharmacological interventions that could be used in people with ID include physiotherapy, massage, cushioning, changing seating position, and applying heat or cold. The effect of pain treatment can be evaluated by self-report but especially by a pain behavior observation checklist appropriate for people with ID and by caregivers who know the characteristic behavior of a specific individual. For healthcare professionals and caregivers, it could be informative to hang up a list in the living facility of the person with ID about specific reactions and interactions when several medications are used simultaneously.

6.7   Conclusion and Recommendation

The current chapter provided a global overview of the challenges that arise in the assessment and treatment of pain in older adults with ID. The complex interplay of medical, pharmacological, cognitive, and communicative factors in this subgroup necessitates further scientific research, literature review, and clinical review of individual cases for a more detailed analysis that is beyond the scope of the chapter. Nonetheless, major themes have been highlighted that include the additional effect of aging on a congenital vulnerability to painful medical conditions and cognitive limitations in self-reporting, the importance of palliative care, and the factors underlying analgesic failure. Nurses should be aware of caregivers' possible misconceptions about pain experience that may arise from atypical pain behavior influenced by the level of ID, learned behavior, and coping style. Therefore, it is recommended that nurses view the pain management of older adults with ID through the total perspective of the history, co-morbidities, and abilities of a person, to be documented in an individual pain profile and pain management plan. Although still prone to difficulties, this method promotes tailor-made assessment and treatment that could also incorporate standardized tools if they are effective for the individual. In conclusion, pain management in people with ID is advancing into a multifaceted approach from personalized medicine, but aging poses new challenges that need to be integrated into the nursing perspective.

References

Ali A, Hassiotis A. Illness in people with intellectual disabilities is common, underdiagnosed, and poorly managed. BMJ. 2008;336:570–1. https://doi.org/10.1136/bmj.39506.386759.80.

American Psychiatric Association. Diagnostic and statistical manual of mental disorders. 5th ed. Arlington: American Psychiatric Association; 2013.

Beacroft M, Dodd K. Pain in people with learning disabilities in residential settings – the need for change. Br J Learn Disabil. 2010;38:201–9.

Biersdorff KK. Incidence of significantly altered pain experience among individuals with developmental disabilities. Am J Ment Retard. 1994;98:619–31.

Bittles AH, Petterson BA, Sullivan SG, Hussain R, Glasson EJ, Montgomery PD. The influence of intellectual disability on life expectancy. J Gerontol Med Sci. 2002;57A:470–2.

Böhmer CJM, Klinkenberg-Knol EC, Niezen-de Boer MC, Meuwissen SGM. Gastroesophageal reflux disease in intellectually disabled individuals: how often, how serious, how manageable? Am J Gastroenterol. 2000;95:1868–72.

Breau LM, MacLaren J, McGrath PJ, Camfield CS, Finley GA. Caregivers' beliefs regarding pain in children with cognitive impairment: relation between pain sensation and reaction increases with severity of impairment. Clin J Pain. 2003;19:335–44.

Buffum MD, Hutt E, Chang VT, Craine MH, Snow AL. Cognitive impairment and pain management: review of issues and challenges. J Rehabil Res Dev. 2007;44:315. https://doi.org/10.1682/JRRD.2006.06.0064.

Canning J, Bandyopadhyay S, Biswas P, Aslund M. Meeting the end of life needs of older adults with intellectual disabilities. In: Chang PE, editor. Contemporary and innovative practice in palliative care. Rijeka: InTech Published; 2012. p. 255–70.

Coppus AMW. People with intellectual disability: what do we know about adulthood and life expectancy? Dev Disabil Res Rev. 2013;18:6–16. https://doi.org/10.1002/ddrr.1123.

Courtenay K, Jokinen NS, Strydom A. Caregiving and adults with intellectual disabilities affected by dementia. J Policy Pract Intellect Disabil. 2010;7:26–33.

De Knegt NC, Pieper MJC, Lobbezoo F, Schuengel C, Evenhuis HM, Passchier J, et al. Behavioral pain indicators in people with intellectual disabilities: a systematic review. J Pain. 2013;14:885–96. https://doi.org/10.1016/j.jpain.2013.04.016.

Defrin R, Pick CG, Peretz C, Carmeli E. A quantitative somatosensory testing of pain threshold in individuals with mental retardation. Pain. 2004;108:58–66. https://doi.org/10.1016/j.pain.2003.12.003.

Defrin R, Lotan M, Pick CG. The evaluation of acute pain in individuals with cognitive impairment: a differential effect of the level of impairment. Pain. 2006;124:312–20. https://doi.org/10.1016/j.pain.2006.04.031.

Devarakonda KM, Lowthian D, Raghavendra T. A case of Rett syndrome with reduced pain sensitivity. Pediatr Anesth. 2009;19:625–7. https://doi.org/10.1111/j.1460-9592.2009.03018.x.

Doody O, Bailey ME. Interventions in pain management for persons with an intellectual disability. J Intellect Disabil. 2017a:174462951770867. https://doi.org/10.1177/1744629517708679.

Doody O, Bailey ME. Pain and pain assessment in people with intellectual disability: issues and challenges in practice. Br J Learn Disabil. 2017b;45:157–65. https://doi.org/10.1111/bld.12189.

Downs J, Géranton SM, Bebbington A, Jacoby P, Bahi-Buisson N, Ravine D, et al. Linking *MECP2* and pain sensitivity: the example of Rett syndrome. Am J Med Genet Part A. 2010;152A:1197–205. https://doi.org/10.1002/ajmg.a.33314.

Evenhuis H, Henderson CM, Beange H, Lennox N, Chicoine B. Healthy aging – adults with intellectual disabilities: physical health issues. J Appl Res Intellect Disabil. 2001;14:175–94.

Ferri R, Musumeci SA, Elia M, Del Gracco S, Scuderi C, Bergonzi P. BIT-mapped somatosensory evoked potentials in the fragile X syndrome. Neurophysiol Clin. 1994;24:413–26.

Findlay L, Williams ACDC, Baum S, Scior K. Caregiver experiences of supporting adults with intellectual disabilities in pain. J Appl Res Intellect Disabil. 2015;28:111–20.

Hennequin M, Faulks D, Veyrune J-L, Bourdiol P. Significance of oral health in persons with Down syndrome: a literature review. Dev Med Child Neurol. 1999;41:275–83.

Hermans H, Evenhuis HM. Multimorbidity in older adults with intellectual disabilities. Res Dev Disabil. 2014;35:776–83. https://doi.org/10.1016/j.ridd.2014.01.022.

Herr K, Coyne PJ, McCaffery M, Manworren R, Merkel S. Pain assessment in the patient unable to self-report: position statement with clinical practice recommendations. Pain Manag Nurs. 2011;12:230–50. https://doi.org/10.1016/j.pmn.2011.10.002.

Jancar J, Speller CJ. Fatal intestinal obstruction in the mentally handicapped. J Intellect Disabil Res. 1994;38:413–22.

Kerr D, Cunningham C, Wilkinson H. Responding to the pain experiences of people with a learning difficulty and dementia. New York: Joseph Rowntree Foundation; 2006.

De Knegt NC, Scherder EJA. Pain in adults with intellectual disabilities. Pain. 2011;152:971–4. https://doi.org/10.1016/j.pain.2010.11.001.

Krigger KW. Cerebral palsy: an overview. Am Fam Physician. 2006;73(1):91–100.

Lauer E, McCallion P. Mortality of people with intellectual and developmental disabilities from select US state disability service systems and medical claims data. J Appl Res Intellect Disabil. 2015;28:394–405.

Lotan M, Moe-nilssen R, Ljunggren AE, Strand LI. Reliability of the non-communicating adult pain checklist (NCAPC), assessed by different groups of health workers. Res Dev Disabil. 2009;30:735–45.

Lotan M, Moe-Nilssen R, Ljunggren AE, Strand LI. Research in developmental disabilities measurement properties of the non-communicating adult pain checklist (NCAPC): a pain scale for adults with intellectual and developmental disabilities, scored in a clinical setting. Res Dev Disabil. 2010;31:367–75.

McCallion P, McCarron M. Ageing and intellectual disabilities: a review of recent literature. Curr Opin Psychiatry. 2004;17:349–52. https://doi.org/10.1097/01.yco.0000139968.14695.95.

McGuire BE, Defrin R. Pain perception in people with Down syndrome: a synthesis of clinical and experimental research. Front Behav Neurosci. 2015;9:1–8. https://doi.org/10.3389/fnbeh.2015.00194.

McGuire B, Daly P, Smyth F. Chronic pain in people with an intellectual disability: under-recognised and under-treated? J Intellect Disabil Res. 2010;54:240–5. https://doi.org/10.1111/j.1365-2788.2010.01254.x.

Miller L, Angulo M, Price D. MR of the pituitary in patients with Prader-Willi syndrome: size determination and imaging findings. Pediatr Radiol. 1996;26:43–7.

Oberlander T, Symons F. Pain in children & adults with developmental disabilities. Baltimore: Paul H. Brooks Publishing Co; 2006.

Paladini A, Fusco M, Coaccioli S, Skaper SD, Varrassi G. Chronic pain in the elderly: the case for new therapeutic strategies. Pain Physician. 2015;18:E863–76.

Patja K, Iivanainen M, Vesala H, Oksanen H, Ruoppila I. Life expectancy of people with intellectual disability: a 35-year follow-up study. J Intellect Disabil Res. 2000;44:591–9.

Priano L, Miscio G, Grugni G, Milano E, Baudo S, Sellitti L, et al. On the origin of sensory impairment and altered pain perception in Prader-Willi syndrome: a neurophysiological study. Eur J Pain. 2009;13:829–35. https://doi.org/10.1016/j.ejpain.2008.09.011.

Price T, Rashid M, Millecamps M, Sanoja R, Entrena J, Cervero F. Decreased nociceptive sensitization in mice lacking the fragile X mental retardation protein. J Neurosci. 2007;27(51): 13958–67.

Reid MC, Bennett DA, Chen WG, Eldadah BA, Farrar JT, Ferrell B, et al. Improving the pharmacologic management of pain in older adults: identifying the research. Pain. 2011;12(9): 1336–57.

Schwartz L, Engel JM, Jensen MP. Pain in persons with cerebral palsy. Arch Phys Med Rehabil. 1999;80:1243–6.

Sheehan R, Ali A, Hassiotis A. Dementia in intellectual disability. Curr Opin Psychiatry. 2014;27:143–8. https://doi.org/10.1097/YCO.0000000000000032.

Sinnema M, Maaskant MA, van Schrojenstein Lantman-de Valk HMJ, Boer H, Curfs LMG, Schrander-Stumpel CTRM. The use of medical care and the prevalence of serious illness in an adult Prader-Willi syndrome cohort. Eur J Med Genet. 2013;56:397–403. https://doi.org/10.1016/j.ejmg.2013.05.011.

Solodiuk JC, Scott-Sutherland J, Meyers M, Myette B, Shusterman C, Karian VE, et al. Validation of the Individualized Numeric Rating Scale (INRS): a pain assessment tool for nonverbal children with intellectual disability. Pain. 2010;150:231–6. https://doi.org/10.1016/j.pain.2010.03.016.

Symons FJ, Shinde SK, Gilles E. Perspectives on pain and intellectual disability. J Intellect Disabil Res. 2008;52:275–86. https://doi.org/10.1111/j.1365-2788.2007.01037.x.

Tuffrey-Wijne I, McEnhill L. Communication difficulties and intellectual disability in end-of-life care. Int J Palliat Nurs. 2008;14:189–95.

Van der Putten A, Vlaskamp C. Pain assessment in people with profound intellectual and multiple disabilities; a pilot study into the use of the Pain Behaviour Checklist in everyday practice. Res Dev Disabil. 2011;32:1677–84. https://doi.org/10.1016/j.ridd.2011.02.020.

van Schrojenstein Lantman-De Valk HM, Metsemakers JF, Haveman MJ, Crebolder HF. Health problems in people with intellectual disability in general practice: a comparative study. Fam Pract. 2000;17:405–7.

Walsh M, Morrison TG, McGuire BE. Chronic pain in adults with an intellectual disability: prevalence, impact, and health service use based on caregiver report. Pain. 2011;152:1951–7. https://doi.org/10.1016/j.pain.2011.02.031.

Weissman-Fogel I, Roth A, Natan-Raav K, Lotan M. Pain experience of adults with intellectual disabilities – caregiver reports. J Intellect Disabil Res. 2015;59(10):914–24. https://doi.org/10.1111/jir.12194.

Zwakhalen SMG, Van Dongen KAJ, Hamers JPH, Abu-Saad HH. Pain assessment in intellectually disabled people: non-verbal indicators. J Adv Nurs. 2004;45:236–45.

Pain in Critically Ill Older Patients

Marie-Madlen Jeitziner, Béatrice Jenni-Moser,
Thekla Brunkert, and Franziska Zúñiga

Abstract

Pain is a common symptom in patients treated in an intensive care unit (ICU) and can be particularly distressing for older patients. Pain is reported by more than half of the patients treated in an ICU, and up to 75% of all medical and surgical ICU patients report the intensity of their pain as moderate to severe. Extrinsic factors such as medical and nursing treatments, or intrinsic factors such as underlying diseases, are important causes of pain. These factors are often very invasive. This chapter, which focuses on pain in critically ill older patients, shows that treating pain requires an interdisciplinary collaboration, including nurses, physicians, and the other healthcare professionals that are involved in treating patients in the ICU. The entire organization or institution must ensure the establishment of interdisciplinary pain management in order to treat pain adequately. The literature recommends using a numerical rating scale for self-assessment of pain, or a behavioral assessment scale for patients who are unable to express themselves verbally. Patient-oriented, individual treatment goals in terms of pain and analgesia management are shown to be effective in reducing pain. Pharmacological and non-pharmacological treatments help older patients reduce their pain.

M.-M. Jeitziner (✉) · B. Jenni-Moser
Department of Intensive Care Medicine, University Hospital Bern (Inselspital),
University of Bern, Bern, Switzerland
e-mail: Marie-Madlen.Jeitziner@insel.ch; Beatrice.Jenni@insel.ch

T. Brunkert · F. Zúñiga
Department Public Health, PT Institute of Nursing Science, Basel University,
Basel, Switzerland
e-mail: thekla.brunkert@unibas.ch; franziska.zuniga@unibas.ch

© Springer International Publishing AG, part of Springer Nature 2018
G. Pickering et al. (eds.), *Pain Management in Older Adults*, Perspectives in Nursing
Management and Care for Older Adults, https://doi.org/10.1007/978-3-319-71694-7_7

7.1   Introduction

The number of older patients (over 75 years of age) hospitalized in intensive care units (ICUs) is increasing (Guidet et al. 2017). Specific reasons for treating older patients in an ICU include exacerbations of chronic illnesses, new catastrophic health problems, trauma caused by home-related accidents and injuries, accidents outside the home, unplanned or planned surgical procedures, illnesses, and end-of-life situations. Older patients are an extremely heterogeneous group, but share two key characteristics: limited physiological reserves due to aging, and multiple co-morbid (chronic) illnesses that often place them in a vulnerable situation, and older patients hospitalized in ICUs have an increased risk of developing a chronic critical illness (Nelson et al. 2010). Chronic critical illnesses may be associated with profound debilitation, lengthy hospitalization, or permanent dependence on mechanical ventilation and/or other life-sustaining technology. Additionally, chronic critical illnesses are related to long-lasting distressing symptoms such as pain, which require long-term medical and nursing care. Frailty is also an issue for older patients. Frailty, characterized by loss of physical and cognitive reserve, has been shown to closely correlate with the aging process, although frailty and aging are not synonymous. Frailty is associated with higher mortality, disability, cognitive impairment, and a poorer quality of life for those affected (Muscedere et al. 2017). However, progress in medicine, nursing, and healthcare technology has allowed a higher proportion of older patients to survive life-threatening illnesses. What is more, following hospitalization in an ICU, the older patients may be even more fragile.

The primary goal of ICU treatment is to maintain, stabilize, and improve the health status of critically ill patients. Treatment in an ICU, coupled with the underlying medical condition requiring ICU admission, is often accompanied by pain and other unpleasant experiences. Pain is reported by more than half of all patients treated in an ICU (Gélinas 2007; Puntillo et al. 2014), and up to 75% of all medical and surgical ICU patients report a pain intensity that is moderate to severe (Gélinas 2007). Pain may be constant for medical and surgical critically ill patients, present even at rest, in addition to resulting from routine care for surgery, trauma or cancer, and various other procedures. Complications due to pain during the ICU stay can include prolonged weaning, adverse effects on the circulatory system, restricted mobility, and impaired wound healing. These complications may also manifest as psychological symptoms, causing anxiety, sleep disorders, and depressive symptoms. In addition to the complications resulting from inadequate pain treatment, there is also the risk of overdose. Both can contribute to prolonged hospital stays and extended ventilation days, leading to a rise in mortality, and additional overall costs.

Older patients' pain is often caused by underlying conditions such as acute, severe, or chronic illnesses. However, there can also be extrinsic pain, as in procedural pain, brought about by medical and nursing interventions such as turning, central venous catheter insertion, wound care, tracheal suctioning, or other necessary interventions. These painful experiences may be amplified by the ICU environment characterized by noise, frequent exposure to light and over- or under-stimulation.

Pain in the ICU has been studied increasingly throughout the past decades, raising questions about post-ICU burden (Jeitziner et al. 2015a, b). Recent evidence suggests that pain may persist after ICU discharge, with half of the patients developing chronic pain (Battle et al. 2013). Puntillo et al. (2016) have shown that some patients remember pain during their stay in the ICU, although few are able to specifically rate pain associated with interventions. For those able to do so, recalled pain intensity and pain distress scores are significantly greater than when reported during the ICU stay, raising the question of whether pain intensity increases in memories of pain, or if patients in the ICU do not accurately report pain intensity. Exposure to intense pain and stress during medical and nursing treatments could be a risk factor that contributes to the transition from acute to chronic pain. Chronic pain signals a major impairment of the neurological pain system (Kyranou and Puntillo 2012). Sepsis, acute respiratory distress symptoms, unrelieved pain, and older age are risk factors for the transition to chronicity (Kyranou and Puntillo 2012). The chronicity of pain may be prevented by appropriately treating acute pain at an early stage. Insufficiently treated pain has been recognized as a risk factor for post-ICU syndrome, which encompasses new or worsening impairment in physical, cognitive, or mental health status following a critical illness, beyond the acute-care hospitalization. Medical and surgical ICU patients, who recall pain and other traumatic situations personally experienced while in the ICU, have a higher incidence of chronic pain and symptoms of post-traumatic stress disorder.

7.2 Pain Assessment

The most valid and reliable pain assessment is via self-assessment (Barr et al. 2013). Valid pain assessment serves as the foundation for adequate pain management. Current practice guidelines state that pain assessment is challenging throughout the ICU stay (Barr et al. 2013; Baron et al. 2015). ICU patients are a particularly vulnerable group at risk of continuing to experience unrecognizable pain due to the severity of their illness, limited ability to communicate, mechanical ventilation, as well as the level of sedation or analgesia (Barr et al. 2013).

Older patients have additional challenges due to age-related changes in vision, hearing, and cognition. Memory, attention and concentration problems, as well as neuropsychological deficits comparable to the impact of low-level dementia, affect a majority of older patients (Wehler 2011). Additionally, older patients tend to under-report their symptoms, perhaps because they accept or believe their symptoms to be normal signs of aging.

The dimensions of pain provide information about the location, intensity, quality, and duration of the pain. In addition, the dimensions of pain show temporal processes, aggravating and soothing factors, and the effect and significance that pain impacts on everyday life. The dimension of pain intensity is particularly important in the ICU due to the patients' limited communicative abilities. The remaining dimensions of pain such as location, quality, and duration, although not a primary focus for treatment in the acute situation, should be assessed as soon as possible.

The insight gained from assessing the dimensions of pain can provide important information that could have a major influence on the physical and psychological recovery (i.e., information regarding restricted functioning due to pain). It can also elicit preferences and experiences in dealing with pain. This information is most likely available only for older patients who are able to verbally express themselves, or whose family members are able to provide insight into the patient's pain experience. Asking relatives about the patient's pain history, however, when a family member is critically ill, can be problematic. It has been found, in particular with relatives of older patients, that they are less capable of describing symptoms and the patient's living situation than the patient himself. Nevertheless, observations in clinical practice carried out by family members and close friends can help assess changes and provide valuable information. Pain assessments conducted by nurses and physicians are equally important. Nurses, in particular, have a great responsibility due to their continuous presence at the bedside of the older patient. As central caregivers for older patients, they have the task of recognizing and observing the course of pain, as well as observing the response to analgesia and non-pharmacological interventions, and must act accordingly.

Practice guidelines recommend using one-dimensional self-report scales that specifically assess acute pain, such as the Numerical Rating Scale (NRS), for critically ill patients (Barr et al. 2013). Chanques et al. (2010) compared the performance of five self-report pain intensity scales. A 0–10 visually enlarged, vertical laminated NRS was the most valid and feasible method for rating pain intensity in the ICU. The Verbal Rating Scale (VRS) also provides helpful information by describing pain in terms of intensity levels (e.g., 'no pain' to 'strongest imaginable pain'). Clinical experience shows that most older patients need to try out two or three different pain assessment scales to assess their pain. It is important that scales be adapted to account for any problems in using them, such as fonts that are too small to read easily. With the help of these one-dimensional scales, pain intensity should be regularly measured according to need, both at rest and during activities such as coughing or turning. Furthermore, it is important that the scales are simple, quick to use, and easily learned, especially for older patients in an ICU.

Older patients who are unable to use the NRS or VRS but who are able to signal a clear YES or NO response should be able to answer a direct question about pain. In this situation, it is recommended to establish a reliable Yes or No system of pain assessment. If self-report is not possible, a behavioral observation scale may be used. The Behavioral Pain Scale (BPS) and the Critical-Care Pain Observation Tool (CPOT) have been found to be the most valid and reliable for this purpose (Payen et al. 2001; Gélinas and Johnston 2007), in particular when they are used regularly by healthcare professionals trained in administering these scales. The behavioral scales measure pain according to facial expressions, upper extremity movements, muscle tension, and compliance with mechanical ventilation. The Behavioral Pain Scale—not intubated (BPS-NI) is utilized for unconscious or uncooperative patients who are not receiving invasive ventilation. In this case, rather than measuring compliance with the ventilator, pain-related sounds are evaluated. The CPOT also has an assessment for non-invasively ventilated patients. A prerequisite to using the CPOT and the BPS is that the motor activities of the patients are present and their behavior can be observed. This is of concern in particular for older patients who, because of the severity of their illness, may not have enough physical strength to physically move in reaction to pain over an extended period of time. The Pain Assessment in Advanced Dementia Scale (PAINAD) offers the possibility of employing someone who is familiar with the patient to assess pain in patients with pre-existing dementia. The scale consists of observable behaviors: breathing, negative vocalization, facial expression, body language, and response to consolation. The scales enable a standardized description of the condition, provide a basis for decision-making on pain therapy and assist in evaluating the effect of the therapy. The pain scales that have been described primarily provide information about acute pain. Further aspects of pain are not taken into account by these scales, including chronic pain, where the patterns of behavior can be completely different, and often affects older patients concurrently. The pain assessment scales are not able to differentiate between acute and chronic pain with symptoms that manifest themselves differently, which is often the situation for older patients. A good pain history assessment may help to deal with this problem proactively.

Nurses and physicians in clinical practice can also use sympathetic nervous system reactions as pain indicators, including changes in blood pressure and pulse, pupillary reactions, or sweating. It should be remembered, however, that changes in vital signs in older patients are not always pain-specific and should be considered as cues to begin further pain assessment using validated and reliable scales (Payen et al. 2001; Gélinas and Johnston 2007).

In order to interpret the varying aspects of pain in a differentiated manner, the literature proposes considering contextual factors, such as: undergoing painful interventions, the particular medical diagnosis, delirium, depth of sedation, and severity of the disease (Barr et al. 2013; Baron et al. 2015). It is often difficult to differentiate pain from anxiety, restlessness, thirst, or even dyspnea for patients in the ICU. Targeted assessment and management of these co-symptoms is critical to reduce the burden caused by an ICU stay for older patients.

7.3 Pain Management

The goal of intensive care medicine provided today is patient-centered with individual treatment goals. Adequate pain therapy requires routine assessments of the individual pain situation, as well as the creation of an analgesia target. This target should take into account, whenever possible, patient preferences and experiences, the cause of the pain, and evaluations of medications and non-pharmaceutical treatments during the ICU stay. The literature recommends recording the goals of therapy and the amount of pain therapy administered at least once per shift (usually every 8 h) and after each therapy change (Barr et al. 2013; Baron et al. 2015). In the immediate postoperative situation, shorter intervals are recommended. Additionally, management of analgesia includes a standardized documentation of side-effects such as nausea, vomiting, and constipation. Using valid scales such as the NRS or a behavioral observation scale (BPS, CPOT) is essential to avoid medication over-dosing and under-dosing.

Ideally, in order for the patient to actively participate in his pain therapy, he should be alert, and free from pain, anxiety, and delirium (Baron et al. 2015; Vincent et al. 2016). The older patient who understands the relevance of manifestations of pain can often have a positive effect on avoiding the progression of his/her pain.

Delirium may pose a dangerous threat for older patients. Older patients are among the group at greatest risk for developing delirium. Delirium has significant consequences for recovery and outcome in the ICU. Delirious, agitated patients often suffer from pain, but are frequently (over-)sedated because of their delirious state. Sedation changes the possible pain-related reactions; thus, the level of sedation is important to consider in order to provide safe and effective pain management. To determine the depth of sedation, a specific scale can be used. The Richmond Agitation Sedation Scale (RASS) is currently used to monitor sedation depth (Barr et al. 2013). Deep sedation is to be avoided whenever possible as it is associated with increased mortality and prolonged ventilation time coupled with an extended ICU stay (Barr et al. 2013). Current treatment strategies should target increasing patient comfort through patient-centered care without excessive sedation. eCASH, meaning "early Comfort using Analgesia, minimal Sedatives and maximal Human care," can ensure that these strategies are implemented in clinical practice. Effective pain relief is therefore the first priority in implementing the strategy of limited sedation. Including family members and friends in caring for the patient also has a major influence on the possibility of reducing sedation (Vincent et al. 2016).

Worldwide, ICUs are implementing evidence-based 'care bundles' (Barr et al. 2013; Morandi et al. 2017). One of the most widely used care bundles is the ABCDEF care bundle, which stands for Awakening and Breathing coordination of daily sedation and ventilator removal trials; Choice of sedative or analgesic exposure; Delirium monitoring and management; Early mobility and exercise and Family-centered care (including the family). The ABCDEF care bundle includes multidisciplinary evidence-based practices that have been shown to improve outcomes for patients in ICUs. The care bundles include multiple complex interventions to assess and manage pain, anxiety, and delirium (Morandi et al. 2017). Significant improvements in patient care in ICUs were shown when the ABCDEF bundle was successfully implemented. The bundle steers the focus of care to all relevant co-symptoms and not only on pain. The care bundle process guides the administration of sedatives and analgesics, mechanical ventilation, and avoidance of immobility, among other measures. Furthermore, families can provide valuable contributions to caring for the patients. The patients recognize their family and feel supported by their family (Morandi et al. 2017). The processes are managed in close cooperation of a multidisciplinary team including nurses, physicians, and physical therapists, ensuring that all interventions focusing on reducing pain, anxiety, delirium, and weakness are interprofessional.

An interprofessional approach to manage and evaluate pain is a key factor in successfully implementing pharmacological and non-pharmacological pain treatments. Although the literature discusses various active pharmacological agents for pain management, opioids remain the primary drug of choice. The selection and use of the appropriate analgesic is further complicated in older persons, as metabolism and drug elimination are often influenced by numerous factors such as altered liver and kidney function. In addition, the method of application is of consideration. Ideally, the drugs should be administered orally, intravenously, or by gavage in the elderly.

Non-pharmacological treatments are complementary to drug-based pain therapy, and include early mobilization, respiratory therapy, physical and occupational therapy, hand massage, positioning, and music therapy. By including the preferences and experiences of patients and their families, one increases the chance that the interventions will be effective. In addition, adapting the treatment environment to reduce stress through noise reduction, initiation of a normal sleep-wake rhythm, and measures to support the patient's orientation are also of value. Reorientation methods within the highly technical environment of the ICU include the earliest possible use of the patient's own vision and hearing aids, targeted communication, daylight, human contact, and various supports such as a clock and a calendar that are easily read and seen, a computer, newspapers, photos, etc. (Gélinas et al. 2013).

Managing pain in older patients requires that nurses and physicians have relevant knowledge about pain management, good communication skills, and professional competence, cooperation, and coordination in interprofessional teams. In addition, one needs a willingness to implement the newest evidence into clinical practice, knowing that older patients and their families must be involved. Nurses, in particular, assume a great responsibility. Their presence ensures that pain management programs are consistent throughout the ICU. Furthermore, older patients are exposed daily to a multitude of procedures that can cause and/or relieve pain. These include turning, moving, or endotracheal aspiration. Prior to initiating these painful interventions, targeted care planning needs to be made including choice of intervention and timing of interventions. For this coordinated decision-making to take place, the organization or institution must support an interprofessional pain management program for older patients.

Conclusion

Pain in older patients hospitalized in an ICU is a significant problem. This fragile patient group needs professionally competent interprofessional pain management to prevent pain from becoming an additional burden in the treatment environment of the ICU. Nursing professionals play an important and central role in interdisciplinary pain management as they often spend extensive time with the older patients and families and know them well.

References

Baron R, Binder A, Biniek R, Braune S, Buerkle H, Dall P, Demirakca S, Eckardt R, Eggers V, Eichler I, Fietze I, Freys S, Fründ A, Garten L, Gohrbandt B, Harth I, Hartl W, Heppner HJ, Horter J, Huth R, Janssens U, Jungk C, Kaeuper KM, Kessler P, Kleinschmidt S, Kochanek M, Kumpf M, Meiser A, Mueller A, Orth M, Putensen C, Roth B, Schaefer M, Schaefers R, Schellongowski P, Schindler M, Schmitt R, Scholz J, Schroeder S, Schwarzmann G, Spies C, Stingele R, Tonner P, Trieschmann U, Tryba M, Wappler F, Waydhas C, Weiss B, Weisshaar G. Evidence and consensus based guideline for the management of delirium, analgesia, and sedation in intensive care medicine. Revision 2015 (DAS-Guideline 2015) - short version. Ger Med Sci. 2015;13:Doc19.

Barr J, Fraser GL, Puntillo K, Ely EW, Gélinas C, Dasta JF, Davidson JE, Devlin JW, Kress JP, Joffe AM, Coursin DB, Herr DL, Tung A, Robinson BR, Fontaine DK, Ramsay MA, Riker RR, Sessler CN, Pun B, Skrobik Y, Jaeschke R. Clinical practice guidelines for the management of pain, agitation, and delirium in adult patients in the intensive care unit. Crit Care Med. 2013;41(1):263–306.

Battle CE, Lovett S, Hutchings H. Chronic pain in survivors of critical illness: a retrospective analysis of incidence and risk factors. Crit Care. 2013;17(3):R101.

Chanques G, Viel E, Constantin JM, Jung B, de Lattre S, Carr J, Cissé M, Lefrant JY, Jaber S. The measurement of pain in intensive care unit: comparison of 5 self-report intensity scales. Pain. 2010;151(3):711–21.

Gélinas C. Management of pain in cardiac surgery ICU patients. Have we improved over time? Intensive Crit Care Nurs. 2007;23(5):298–303.

Gélinas C, Johnston C. Pain assessment in the critically ill ventilated adult: validation of the critical-care pain observation tool and physiologic indicators. Clin J Pain. 2007;23(6):497–505.

Gélinas C, Arbour C, Michaud C, Robar L, Côté J. Patients and ICU nurses' perspectives of non-pharmacological interventions for pain management. Nurs Crit Care. 2013;18(6):307–18.

Guidet B, Leblanc G, Simon T, Woimant M, Quenot JP, Ganansia O, Maignan M, Yordanov Y, Delerme S, Doumenc B, Fartoukh M, Charestan P, Trognon P, Galichon B, Javaud N, Patzak A, Garrouste-Orgeas M, Thomas C, Azerad S, Pateron D, Boumendil A. Effect of systematic intensive care unit triage on long-term mortality among critically ill elderly patients in France: a randomized clinical trial. JAMA. 2017;318(15):1450–9.

Jeitziner MM, Hamers JP, Bürgin R, Hantikainen V, Zwakhalen SM. Long-term consequences of pain, anxiety and agitation for critically ill older patients after an intensive care unit stay. J Clin Nurs. 2015a;24(17-18):2419–28.

Jeitziner MM, Zwakhalen SM, Bürgin R, Hantikainen V, Hamers JP. Changes in health-related quality of life in older patients one year after an intensive care unit stay. J Clin Nurs. 2015b;24(21-22):3107–17.

Kyranou M, Puntillo K. The transition from acute to chronic pain: might intensive care unit patients be at risk? Ann Intensive Care. 2012;2(1):36.

Morandi A, Piva S, Ely EW, Myatra SN, Salluh JIF, Amare D, Azoulay E, Bellelli G, Csomos A, Fan E, Fagoni N, Girard TD, Heras La Calle G, Inoue S, Lim CM, Kaps R, Kotfis K, Koh Y, Misango D, Pandharipande PP, Permpikul C, Cheng Tan C, Wang DX, Sharshar T, Shehabi Y, Skrobik Y, Singh JM, Slooter A, Smith M, Tsuruta R, Latronico N. Worldwide Survey of the "assessing pain, both spontaneous awakening and breathing trials, choice of drugs, delirium monitoring/management, early exercise/mobility, and family empowerment" (ABCDEF) bundle. Crit Care Med. 2017;45(11):e1111–22.

Muscedere J, Waters B, Varambally A, Bagshaw SM, Boyd JG, Maslove D, Sibley S, Rockwood K. The impact of frailty on intensive care unit outcomes: a systematic review and meta-analysis. Intensive Care Med. 2017;43(8):1105–22.

Nelson JE, Cox CE, Hope AA, Carson SS. Chronic critical illness. Am J Respir Crit Care Med. 2010;182(4):446–54.

Payen JF, Bru O, Bosson JL, Lagrasta A, Novel E, Deschaux I, Lavagne P, Jacquot C. Assessing pain in critically ill sedated patients by using a behavioral pain scale. Crit Care Med. 2001;29(12):2258–63.

Puntillo KA, Max A, Timsit JF, Vignoud L, Chanques G, Robleda G, Roche-Campo F, Mancebo J, Divatia JV, Soares M, Ionescu DC, Grintescu IM, Vasiliu IL, Maggiore SM, Rusinova K, Owczuk R, Egerod I, Papathanassoglou ED, Kyranou M, Joynt GM, Burghi G, Freebairn RC, Ho KM, Kaarlola A, Gerritsen RT, Kesecioglu J, Sulaj MM, Norrenberg M, Benoit DD, Seha MS, Hennein A, Periera FJ, Benbenishty JS, Abroug F, Aquilina A, Monte JR, An Y, Azoulay E. Determinants of procedural pain intensity in the intensive care unit: the European® study. Am J Respir Crit Care Med. 2014;189(1):39–47.

Puntillo KA, Max A, Chaize M, Chanques G, Azoulay E. Patient recollection of ICU procedural pain and post ICU Burden: the memory study. Crit Care Med. 2016;44(11):1988–95.

Vincent JL, Shehabi Y, Walsh TS, Pandharipande PP, Ball JA, Spronk P, Longrois D, Strøm T, Conti G, Funk GC, Badenes R, Mantz J, Spies C, Takala J. Comfort and patient-centred care without excessive sedation: the eCASH concept. Intensive Care Med. 2016;42(6):962–71.

Wehler M. Long-term outcome of elderly patients after intensive care treatment. Med Klin Intensivmed Notfmed. 2011;106(1):29–33.

Nursing Roles in Managing Pain in Older Adults

Abby Wickson-Griffiths, Sharon Kaasalainen, and Laura Pokoradi

Abstract

As the global population continues to age (National Institutes of Health, Global health and aging [Report on the internet] http://www.who.int/ageing/publications/global_health.pdf, 2011), direct care practitioners, researchers, and policy makers, including nurses, must work together to engage older adults in identifying and managing health concerns. Although sometimes mistakenly attributed to the aging process (Coker et al., Appl Nurs Res 23:139–46, 2010), pain is common in older adults, who can experience multiple modes of pain including acute, persistent (chronic), postoperative, neuropathic, and cancer (Cavalieri, J Am Osteopath Assoc 105:S12–17, 2005). Key challenges to managing pain in older adults have been attributed to an increased risk for adverse effects from pharmacological treatments, presence of comorbidities, polypharmacy, multimodal pain presentation, poor reporting of pain for older adults, as well as poor pain management strategies employed by the healthcare professionals (Wickson-Griffiths et al., Clin Geriatr Med 32:693–704, 2016). Given these complex challenges, pain in older adults is ideally managed by an interdisciplinary team of healthcare professionals, an approach, which has been supported in the pain literature and through expert opinion (Wickson-Griffiths et al., Clin Geriatr Med 32:693–704, 2016; Hadjistavropoulos et al., Clin J Pain 2:S1–43, 2007). One of the key roles

A. Wickson-Griffiths (✉)
Faculty of Nursing, University of Regina, Regina, SK, Canada
e-mail: abigail.wickson-griffiths@uregina.ca

S. Kaasalainen
McMaster University School of Nursing, Hamilton, ON, Canada
e-mail: kaasal@mcmaster.ca

L. Pokoradi
Hamilton Health Sciences, Hamilton, ON, Canada
e-mail: pokorlau@HHSC.CA

© Springer International Publishing AG, part of Springer Nature 2018
G. Pickering et al. (eds.), *Pain Management in Older Adults*, Perspectives in Nursing Management and Care for Older Adults, https://doi.org/10.1007/978-3-319-71694-7_8

on the interdisciplinary team is that of the nurse, who will contribute to managing client pain.

While there may be differences in nurses' legislated scope of practice, they are accountable for ensuring that their clients presenting with pain have effective assessment and management (Burns and McIlfatrick, Int J Palliative Nurs 21:400–7, 2015). Based on their holistic assessment of the client, nurses can offer prescribed medical or nursing pain intervention and monitor for its effectiveness, as well as advocate for and coordinate pain management (Burns and McIlfatrick, Int J Palliative Nurs 21:400–7, 2015). Accordingly, this chapter will describe common international nursing roles, setting the context for nurses' suitability to manage pain in older adults. Next, guidelines and directives that nurses can incorporate into their practice will be highlighted and described. Subsequently, the nursing role in pain management with older adults will be explored, with special attention to the community and long-term care context. Finally, future directions including more resources to support nurses in managing pain will be listed and described.

8.1 Description of Nursing Roles

In order to better understand the position of the nurse in managing pain, this section will briefly describe the definition of a nurse as well as three internationally recognized nursing titles, including the licensed practical, registered, and advanced practice nurse according to their educational preparation as well as general scope of practice. It is important to note that while there is encouragement to work toward a global standard in nurse education, there is *great international diversity* in nursing educational preparation as well as regulation and practice (Institute of Medicine 2011). Given the variability of nursing practice, examples that are specific to Canadian nurses will be given for a frame of reference.

The International Council of Nurses (2017) defines a nurse as:

"… a person who has completed a program of basic, generalized nursing education and is authorized by the appropriate regulatory authority to practice nursing in his/her country… The nurse is prepared and authorized (National Institutes of Health 2011) to engage in the general scope of nursing practice, including the promotion of health, prevention of illness, and care of physically ill, mentally ill, and disabled people of all ages and in all health care and other community settings; (Coker et al. 2010) to carry out health care teaching; (Cavalieri 2005) to participate fully as a member of the health care team; (Wickson-Griffiths et al. 2016) to supervise and train nursing and health care auxiliaries; and (Hadjistavropoulos et al. 2007) to be involved in research."

Registered nurses (RNs) have passed both a board/council-approved initial nursing education program (usually 36–48 months) and an entry-to-practice examination (where required) (International Council of Nurses (ICN) 2011). Many countries now require a baccalaureate degree as a minimum educational requirement; however, this is not universal. In addition, the RNs must continue to meet the standards or competencies of the nursing board (provincial/state or national) through continual licensure, where required ((ICN) 2011). In Canada, RNs require a baccalaureate degree as well as have the capacity to demonstrate entry-level competencies for knowledge, skills, and judgment (Canadian Nurses Association (CNA) 2015). While each Canadian province regulates the registered nurses' scope of practice, RNs provide direct client care as well as organize care and support clients of all ages in managing their health concerns. In addition to direct client care, RNs engage in education, research, and administration activities in a variety of care and home settings ((CNA) 2015).

Licensed practical nurses (LPNs) have also passed both a board/council-approved initial nursing education program (usually 12–24 months) and an entry-to-practice exam (Canadian Institute for Health Information (CIHI) 2017). LPNs in Canada must demonstrate entry-level competencies related to knowledge, skill, and judgment (Canadian Council for Practical Nurse Regulators (CCPNR) 2013). Like RNs, LPNs are accountable for their nursing actions and practice in a variety of health and home care settings ((CCPNR) 2013). While there is overlap in the practice of LPNs and RNs, both types of nurses can care for clients that have been assessed to be less complex and have a lower risk for negative health outcome. However, RNs would be more involved in the care of more complex patients requiring more needs to be met ((CNA) 2015).

Advanced practice nurses' (CNA 2009) roles are being developed internationally; however, International Council of Nurses defines the following:

"A Nurse Practitioner (NP)/Advanced Practice Nurse is a registered nurse who has acquired the expert knowledge base, complex decision-making skills and clinical competencies for expanded practice, the characteristics of which are shaped by the context and/or country in which s/he is credentialed to practice. A master's degree is recommended for entry level."

In Canada, generally, NPs can "autonomously diagnose, order and interpret diagnostic tests, prescribe pharmaceuticals and perform specific procedures within their legislated scope of practice" (CNA 2009). However, not all APNs are NPs, requiring specific provincial legislation for a skill set beyond the scope of the RN (CNA 2007). Nurses with a minimum graduate-level education, with advanced clinical and leadership skills, may practice as an APN, using employer-driven titles such as APN, clinical nurse specialist, nurse specialist, or educator titles (Musclow et al. 2002).

In all, nurses have the educational preparation as well as continuing accountability to clients and practice through maintaining their licensure (where required). They have capability to participate as a healthcare team member through direct client, education, and research.

8.2   Pain Management Guidance for Nurses

As noted, nurses are key players within the interdisciplinary team to provide pain management care to the older adult. To help guide care from a nursing perspective, the following section provides selected guidelines and directives related to pain management in:

- Evidence-based approaches for the interdisciplinary team, including nurses
- Approaches and competencies for nurses
- Nursing care of the older adult

8.3   Evidence-Based Guidelines for Managing Pain in Older Adults

Pain management in older adult is complex, which required the establishment of guidelines specific to types of pain and treatment in this population. It is noted that pain education and guidelines are varied in for this population (Schofield 2012). The following provides examples of evidence-based guidelines that nurses as well other healthcare providers can use to inform their practice in the care of older adults.

- American Geriatrics Society Panel on Pharmacological Management of Persistent Pain in Older Persons (USA) (American Geriatrics Society Panel on Pharmacological Management of Persistent Pain in Older Persons 2009)
- Evidence-Based Practice Guideline: Acute Pain Management in Older Adults[1] (USA) (Cornelius et al. 2017)
- Evidence-Based Practice Guideline: Persistent Pain Management in Older Adults (see footnote 1) (USA) (Arnstein et al. 2017)

8.4   Selected Guidance for Nurses Managing Pain

In addition to the evidence-based guidelines for specific pain and treatment, nurses may also seek out direction from their regulatory body or professional practice association for publications specific to pain management nursing. The following are two examples from a professional college (UK) and association (Canada) that provide nurses with detailed information around pain management nursing competencies and guidelines specific to the nursing process, respectively.

Endorsed by the British Pain Society, the Royal College of Nursing (2015) produced the *Pain Knowledge and Skills Framework for the Nursing Team*, based on

---

[1] Note that the guidelines published in the *Journal of Gerontological Nursing* are condensed versions available to purchase through the Csomay Center for Gerontological Excellence.

the initial framework created by the Nurses' Interest Group of the New Zealand Pain Society in 2013. The framework, produced by a regulatory body, outlines the pain management competencies for unregulated and regulated nursing care providers, with progressive degrees of expertise. Highlights include:

- Unregistered staff and registered nurses can use the detailed competencies, according to their level of expertise, to reflect on and develop their knowledge, skills, and confidence in managing pain in varying populations.
- Nursing leadership can use the competencies as a guide to help mentor nurses' effectiveness in managing pain and plan for education components in practice.

The Registered Nurses' Association of Ontario (RNAO 2013), a provincial nursing association, has developed a series of *Best Practice Guidelines* for nurses on topics such as the prevention and/or management of health conditions, promoting safety, and approaches to care. The *Assessment and Management of Pain (3rd Ed)* is included in this series and offers nurses evidence-based approaches to pain assessment, planning, implementation of a pain management plan, and evaluation of pain management interventions. In addition, recommendations for education and organization and policy are included for nursing leadership consideration. Highlights include:

- Recommendations for nursing practice are supported with levels of evidence from the literature (e.g., meta-analysis, experimental study, expert opinion panel).
- Specific resources for pain assessment tools for specific populations including children and older adults are included as appendices.

8.5 Selected Guidance for Nurses Managing Pain in Older Adults

The National Guideline Clearinghouse makes *Pain Management in Older Adults: In Evidence-Based Geriatric Nursing Protocols for Best Practice* (Horgas et al. 2012) available for nurses. This concise, evidence-based guideline includes recommendations for strategies in pain assessment, nursing care, and treatment that are specific to older adults.

- This guideline provides links to companion documents around pain assessment in the older adult through the Hartford Institute for Geriatric Nursing website.
- Like the RNAO document, this guideline provides readers with the level of evidence from the literature in the recommendations for practice.

MacSorley and colleagues (2014) provide specific guidance to hospice and home care nurses caring for older adults through their publication *Pain Assessment and*

Management Strategies for Elderly Patients. The article provides strategies to this subset of nurses through approaches to pain assessment and communication within the interdisciplinary team. Highlights include:

- The MacSorley Communication Model: Elderly Pain Model, which captures key elements caring for older adults and their family caregivers, as well as communicating within the interdisciplinary team. The role of the home healthcare nurse in assessing for and managing pain, including patient and family education, is specifically highlighted.
- This article also captures relevant pain medications and considerations in the older adult.

8.6 Highlight on Nursing Roles in Pain Management in Older Adults

This section will provide examples of how nurses are involved in managing pain in older adults. As noted, nurses practice through direct patient care, education, research, and administration (Canadian Nurses Association (CNA) 2015) and can involve pain management considerations in each of these domains. Nurses can provide direct care through noticing and assessing pain, implementing a plan of care, and monitoring and evaluating effect of intervention (American Geriatrics Society Panel on Pharmacological Management of Persistent Pain in Older Persons 2009). They are involved in providing direct patient pain care to persons of all ages, including older adults in a variety of settings including the community/clinic, hospital and long-term care (Musclow et al. 2002; Courtenay and Carey 2008; Kaasalainen et al. 2010). Registered nurses, and especially advanced practice nurses, with expert knowledge, are well-positioned to provide education and consultation for both patients and staff (Musclow et al. 2002; Kaasalainen et al. 2010, 2015). Graduate-level nurses have taken a keen interest in evaluating the role of the nurse in pain management (Kaasalainen et al. 2016), synthesizing bodies of research related to pain management nursing and/or creating practice guidelines (Tsai et al. 2017). Finally, nurse administrators can work in collaboration with nurses and other healthcare providers to effect policy and procedural changes within their facility.

As noted, registered and advanced practice nurses work in a variety of settings, helping to manage pain for patients of all ages including older adults. The following provides examples of nurses working directly with older adults and staff in efforts to manage pain in the community and long-term care contexts.

8.7   Registered Nurses Working with Older Adults in the Community

Box 8.1 Highlight on Nurses Working in the Community or Clinic with Older Adults
Context:

- There has been significant interest in older adults "aging in place," with primary care being provided in the community in favor of residential-based care (Wiles et al. 2011).
- At least 25% (up to an estimated 76%) of older adults living in the community experience persistent pain, with up to 46% experiencing current pain (Abdulla et al. 2013).
- Nurses may lead pain management strategies in the community with their interdisciplinary counterparts to help relieve pain for community-dwelling older adults.

Highlight roles in pain management:

- Along with other ailments, home healthcare nurses help older adults to manage pain related to osteoarthritis (Kee and Epps 2001). Kee and Epps' (Kee and Epps 2001) qualitative study explored registered nurses' roles in promoting pain management to older adults with osteoarthritis. Through a thematic content analysis, authors reported that registered nurses promoted pain management through *understanding pain* by *knowing how to assess* and *knowing about pain treatment*s. Registered nurses shared the importance of knowing and evaluating older adults' medications as well as trying non-pharmacological treatments such as distraction, heat, and exercise as complementary therapies. Authors also identified the theme of *wanting to provide good nursing care* through *trying but frustrated* and *needing more knowledge*. Registered nurses tried their best strategies to help relieve pain, however, could feel frustrated when this outcome was not achieved.
- Muntinga and colleagues (Muntinga et al. 2016) investigated how practice nurse-led, in-home, comprehensive geriatric assessments might improve pain care for older adults in the Netherlands. Working within

the Geriatric Care Model, practice nurses completed assessments, arranged for supported services for the older adult, and organized and participated in multidisciplinary consultations with other team members (e.g., geriatric expert team, physician, and pharmacist). Practice nurses identified new cases of pain (10.6% of participants), and the majority of these older adults wanted a tailored pain care plan, which was co-created with the nurse.

Innovation in pain management: In Ontario, Canada, there are pain clinics in the community and in tertiary care centers. The level of complexity of the interventions provided is determined by each care setting. In a community clinic, the nurse prepares medications and admits and discharges patients. This includes documentation, history, and vital signs.

The nursing role is more extensive in a tertiary care pain clinic. There are infusions of lidocaine or ketamine offered, as well as a variety of interventions such as epidurals, stellate ganglion blocks, rhizotomies, facet injection, sacroiliac injections, and lumbar sympathetic blocks (some of which are done under fluoroscopic or ultrasound guidance). Tertiary pain clinic nurses do admission history, which includes the evaluation of previous intervention, medication reconciliation, vital signs, and starting intravenous access. Post-procedure, the patient has vital signs done and is accessed for complications and the IV is discontinued. The RN is in the procedure room, as these patients may have adverse events, thus not considered to have a stable and predictable outcome. For the procedure, the nurse sets up necessary equipment and monitors the patient throughout the procedure, takes vital signs, and gives any needed medications. Patients are able to call nurses for questions about medication or procedures, including concerns about symptoms post-procedures.

The referrals to the clinic are also triaged by nurses, to the appropriate physician and programs. They are triaged to medical or interventional management and possibly to the self-management program if appropriate. There are programs for self-management of pain. These are group based with education on various topics and strategies to manage their pain. In this program nurses facilitate some of those classes.

8.8   Advanced Practice Nurses Working in Long-Term Care Settings

Box 8.2 Highlight on Nurse Practitioners and Clinical Nurse Specialist Working in Long-Term Care
Context:

- Residential long-term care settings can be home to some of society's most older and medically complex adults, most with two or more chronic conditions (Ontario Long-Term Care Association 2016).
- It is estimated that between 83 and 93% of persons residing in facility-based care have persistent pain, with up to 73% having current pain (Abdulla et al. 2013).
- Advanced practice nurses provide direct patient care as well as engage in educational, research, and administrative duties (Canadian Nurses Association (CNA) 2015), which well-positions them to engage in multipronged approaches to managing residents' pain.

Nurse practitioner roles in pain management: As nurse practitioners were introduced in the Canadian long-term care home settings in the 2000s (Stollee et al. 2006), clarity around their pain management role was investigated through self-reporting of their primary activities (Kaasalainen et al. 2007). Nurse practitioners reported either providing pain management or mostly agreed that they should be involved with the following domains of care:

- *Clinical practice:* assessing resident pain, ordering diagnostic tests, diagnosing cause of resident pain, prescribing pharmacological and non-pharmacological treatments, and monitoring for effectiveness and side effects (e.g., analgesics, NSAIDS, opioids from a prescribed list, adjuvant therapies).
- *Consultation and communication:* collaborating with members of the healthcare team, including family members and residents, to manage pain.

- *Education:* providing staff nurses with education and family members and residents with counsel on pain management.
- *Leadership/change agent:* participating in committee work as well as policy and procedures development, liaising with regulatory bodies about pain management activities, and implementing and evaluating pain management programs.
- *Advocacy:* advocating for residents, families, and nursing staff for pain management.
- *Research:* identifying researchable questions, participating in, and disseminating research findings around pain management.

Innovation in pain management: Kaasalainen and colleagues (Kaasalainen et al. 2012, 2015, 2016) have explored the use of the advanced practice nurse (nurse practitioners and clinical nurse specialists) as a "change champion" in implementing evidence-based pain assessment tools and protocols in the long-term care home setting in Canada. In general, change champions were responsible for leading the changes to pain management practices through educational initiatives within an interdisciplinary pain team that they also helped to develop. Nurse practitioners (as well as clinical nurse specialists (Kaasalainen et al. 2012, 2015)) used a variety of strategies to engage the pain team and other long-term care home staff to implement changes to pain practices including contributing to developing the pain management procedure (Kaasalainen et al. 2016), facilitating or arranging for one-on-one and/or in-service pain management education (Kaasalainen et al. 2015, 2016), working with staff to manageably "phase in" new practices (Kaasalainen et al. 2015), reminding staff to practice according to the new protocol (Kaasalainen et al. 2015), providing feedback to staff through reviewing their pain documented practices (Kaasalainen et al. 2015), facilitating interdisciplinary pain team meetings (Kaasalainen et al. 2015, 2016), and creating positive relationships with staff (Kaasalainen et al. 2015). Importantly, implementing an advanced practice nurse-led pain change in practice showed promising results for residents in reducing pain (Kaasalainen et al. 2016) or experiencing less of an increase in pain (Kaasalainen et al. 2012) and improved functional status (Kaasalainen et al. 2016) over the intervention periods when compared to care as usual. In addition, clinical practice at the intervention sites also improved around completing and documenting resident pain assessments (Kaasalainen et al. 2012, 2016), using evidence-based pain assessment tools (Kaasalainen et al. 2012), developing care plans to manage pain, and documenting the effect of pain intervention (Kaasalainen et al. 2016).

8.9   Future Directions

The recognition that pain is under-assessed and managed in the older adult population in a variety of healthcare and home settings (Long 2013) can be a call for
nurses to take action to improve this status quo. As a group, nurses' educational
background coupled with their clinical experience situates them to be key players
on the interdisciplinary team to address the pain management needs of older adults.
This section will highlight current challenges and how nurse education and targeted implementation of programing as well as group engagement can make a
positive impact.

8.10   Challenges, Education, and Implementation
            Directed at Nurses

Although nurses have an important role in managing pain in older adults, they may
lack the knowledge and skill set to be able to always effectively intervene (Long
2013). Study findings from a variety of settings have identified barriers to effective
pain management in older adults (Coker et al. 2010; Burns and McIlfatrick 2015;
Park et al. 2016) through a literature review on nurses' knowledge and attitudes
toward pain management in dementia care that they have challenges in identifying
pain, due to the person with dementia's inability to report it; accessing and using
pain assessment tools; and needing additional training and education. In addition,
while exploring the implementation of a best practice approach in acute medical
units for older adults, Coker and colleagues (2010) found that nurses commonly
reported barriers that interfered with optimal pain management. Registered nurses
identified barriers such as having difficulty in assessing a person with cognitive
impairment, sensory problems, or language barriers, as well as inadequate time to
implement non-pharmacological interventions or teach older adults about pain
management. Also, in the community setting, Park and colleagues (Park et al. 2016)
interviewed nurses working at public health centers who made home visits to low-
income older adults about barriers to managing chronic pain. Nurses reported barriers related to their own limitations in managing chronic pain related to their lacking
knowledge, experience, and confidence. Overall, research findings suggest that
nurses working with older adults in home and healthcare settings have barriers to
overcome as they continue to help relieve pain in this population.

To address barriers and improve nursing capacity to deliver effect pain management to older adults (Long 2013; Long et al. 2010; Tse and Ho 2013), researchers
and clinicians have implemented educational opportunities and programs. The following will highlight some of these efforts in the long-term care home setting. In
addition to the positive impact, advanced practice nurses have been working as

change champions to provide education and consultation to long-term care staff (Kaasalainen et al. 2015, 2016, 2012); others have addressed perceived barriers through:

- Implementing the "Campaign Against Pain," which included both interdisciplinary staff and resident working groups to comprehensively revise pain policy and procedures as well as provide education and expert consultation to improve both direct care and support staff's knowledge, attitudes, and beliefs around pain management (Long 2013; Long et al. 2010)
- Implementing an integrative pain management program, which included 8 weeks of both pain education sessions for nursing staff and leisure instruction for residents, which not only improved nursing knowledge and attitudes but reduced resident pain scores (Tse and Ho 2013)

8.11   Getting and Staying Engaged

Nurses can get and stay involved with pain management from clinical, educational, and research perspectives by joining international, national, and/or local pain interest groups. Collectively, groups may offer exciting opportunities for education through programs, conferences, and resources as well as networking and collaborating within special or shared interest groups. Box 8.3 outlines examples of societies or adults.

Box 8.3 Pain Related Society/Groups
International Association for the Study of Pain (IASP (International Association for the Study of Pain 2017)): https://www.iasp-pain.org/Chapters?navItemNumber=566

- IASP engages stakeholder groups, including healthcare providers, scientists, and policy makers to support the study of pain and disseminate knowledge all over the world.
- IASP has nearly 100 national chapters and 20 pain-related special interest groups.
- Special/Shared Interest Group.
    ◦ Pain in Older Persons: https://www.iasp-pain.org/SIG/OlderPersons.

American Pain Society (APS (American Pain Society 2017)): http://americanpainsociety.org/

- The APS engages clinicians and scientists to create awareness of pain to positively transform practice and policy.
- APS has 17 special interest groups and opportunities to attend educational and networking events.
- Special interest groups related to nursing or older adults.

- o Nursing Shared Interest Group: http://americanpainsociety.org/get-involved/shared-interest-groups/nursing.
- o Geriatric Pain Shared Interest Group: http://americanpainsociety.org/get-involved/shared-interest-groups/geriatric-pain.

American Society for Pain Management Nursing (ASPMN (American Society for Pain Management Nursing 2017)): http://www.aspmn.org/Pages/default.aspx

- • ASPMN promotes optimal pain care through best nursing practices.
- • ASPMN offers educational and certification opportunities for pain management.

The Canadian Pain Society (CPS (The Canadian Pain Society 2017)): http://www.canadianpainsociety.ca/

- • The CPS engages clinicians and scientists with an interest in pain management and research.
- • The CPS has four interest groups and offers opportunities for education and networking.
- • Special/Shared Interest Group.
  - o Nursing Issues Special Interest Group: http://www.canadianpainsociety.ca/?page=NursingIssues.

The Australian Pain Society (AuPS (The Australian Pain Society 2017)): https://www.apsoc.org.au/

- • The AuPS engages multidisciplinary members with the mission of relieving pain and suffering through clinical practice, education, and research.
- • The AuPS has two special interest groups and offers educational resources and networking events.
- • Special/Shared Interest Group.
  - o Nursing Issues Sub-Group: http://www.canadianpainsociety.ca/?page=NursingIssues.

The British Pain Society (BPS (The British Pain Society 2017)): https://www.britishpainsociety.org/

- • The BPS engages multidisciplinary members with the interest of improving pain management.
- • The BPS has 14 pain-related special interest groups and further opportunities for education and networking.
- • Older Adult Special Interest Group: https://www.britishpainsociety.org/pain-in-older-people-special-interest-group/.

Nurses may also engage through their local regulatory body or professional association in pain management groups. Swafford and colleagues (Swafford et al. 2014) offer that nurses may seek out available online pain management resources, some of which may include:

- The University of Iowa's Geriatric Pain site (The University of Iowa 2017): https://geriatricpain.org/
- The Hartford Institute for Geriatric Nursing—ConsultGeri (Hartford Institute for Geriatric Nursing 2017): https://consultgeri.org/
- The Portal of Geriatrics Online Education (ADGAP 2017): http://www.pogoe. org
- The RNAO's Assessment and Management of Pain in the Elderly Learning Package (RNAO 2007): http://rnao.ca/sites/rnao-ca/files/Assessment_and_ Management_of_Pain_in_the_Elderly_-_Learning_Package_for_LTC.pdf

References

Abdulla A, Adams N, Bone M, Elliott AM, Gaffin J, Jones D, et al. Guidance on the management of pain in older people. Age Ageing. 2013;42(1):i1–57.

ADGAP [Internet]. The portal of geriatrics online education. 2017. [cited 18 Dec 2017]. Available from https://www.pogoe.org/.

American Geriatrics Society Panel on Pharmacological Management of Persistent Pain in Older Persons. Pharmacological management of persistent pain in older adults. J Am Geriatr Soc. 2009;57(8):1331–46.

American Pain Society [Internet]. 2017. [cited 18 Dec 2017]. Available from http://americanpain-society.org/.

American Society for Pain Management Nursing [Internet]. 2017. [cited 2017 December 18]. Available from http://www.aspmn.org/Pages/default.aspx.

Arnstein P, Herr K, Butcher H. Evidence-based practice guideline: persistent Pain Management in Older Adults. J Gerontol Nurs. 2017;43(7):20–31.

Burns M, McIlfatrick S. Palliative care in dementia: literature review of nurses' knowledge and attitudes toward pain assessment. Int J Palliat Nurs. 2015;21(8):400–7.

Canadian Council for Practical Nurse Regulators (CCPNR). Entry-to-practice competencies for licensed practical nurses [Document available on the internet]. 2013; [cited 18 Dec 2017]. Available from https://www.clpnbc.org/Documents/Practice-Support-Documents/Entry-to-Practice-Competencies-(EPTC)-LPNs.aspx.

Canadian Institute for Health Information (CIHI). Licensed practical nurses. 2017; [cited 18 Dec 2017]; [about 2 screens]. Available from https://www.cihi.ca/en/licensed-practical-nurses.

Canadian Nurses Association (CNA). Framework for the practice of registered nurses in Canada. 2015 [Document on the internet]. 2015; [cited 18 Dec 2017]. p. 40. Available from https://www.cna-aiic.ca/en/becoming-an-rn/the-practice-of-nursing.

Cavalieri TA. Management of pain in older adults. J Am Osteopath Assoc. 2005;105(3):S12–7.

CNA. Position statement: Advanced practice nursing. 2007; [cited 18 Dec 2017]. Available from https://www.cna-aiic.ca/~/media/cna/page-content/pdf-en/ps60_advanced_nursing_practice_2007_e.pdf?la=en.

CNA. Position statement: the nurse practitioner. 2009; [cited 18 Dec 2017]. Available from https://cna-aiic.ca/~/media/cna/page-content/pdf-fr/ps_nurse_practitioner_e.pdf?la=en.

Coker E, Pappaioannou A, Kaasalainen S, Dolovich L, Turpie I, Taniguchi A. Nurses' perceived barriers to optimal pain management in older adults on acute medical units. Appl Nurs Res. 2010;23:139–46.

Cornelius R, Herr KA, Gordon DB, Kretzer K. Evidence-based practice guideline acute pain Management in Older Adults. J Gerontol Nurs. 2017;43(2):18–27. https://doi.org/10.3928/00989134-20170111-08.

Courtenay M, Carey N. The impact and effectiveness of nurse-led care in the management of acute and chronic pain: a review of the literature. J Clin Nurs. 2008;17:2001–13.

Hadjistavropoulos T, Herr K, Turk DC, Fine PG, Dworkin RH, Helme R, et al. An interdisciplinary expert consensus statement on assessment of pain in older adult. Clin J Pain. 2007;2:S1–43.

Hartford Institute for Geriatric Nursing [Internet]. ConsultGeri. 2017. [cited 18 Dec 2017]. Available from https://consultgeri.org/.

Horgas AL, Yoon SL, Grall M. Pain management in older adults. In: Evidence based geriatric nursing protocols for best practice. [Document available on the internet]. 2012. Available from http://www.guidelines.gov/summar/summary.aspx?ss$^{1/4}$15&doc_id$^{1/4}$10198&string.

Institute of Medicine. The future of nursing: leading change, advancing health [report on the internet]. Washington, DC: The National Academies Press; 2011. p. 620. Note to editors: Information specifically used in paper is from Appendix J. Available from https://www.nap.edu/read/12956/chapter/1.

International Association for the Study of Pain [Internet]. 2017. IASP Chapters; [cited 18 Dec 2017]; [about 2 screens]. Available from https://www.iasp-pain.org/Chapters?navItemNumber=566.

International Council for Nurses. Definition of nursing. 2017; [cited 18 Dec 2017]; [about 1 screen]. Available from http://www.icn.ch/who-we-are/icn-definition-of-nursing/.

International Council of Nurses (ICN). ICN framework of competencies for the generalist nurse. Geneva, Switzerland: 2003. Cited in: The future of nursing: leading change, advancing health [Report on the internet]. Washington, DC: The National Academies Press; 2011. p. 620. Available from https://www.nap.edu/read/12956/chapter/1.

Kaasalainen S, DiCenso A, Donald FC, Staples E. Optimizing the role of the nurse practitioner in improve pain management in long-term care. CJNR. 2007;39(2):14–31.

Kaasalainen S, Martin-Misener R, Carter N, DiCenso A, Donald F, Baxter P. The nurse practitioner role in pain management in long-term care. J Adv Nurs. 2010;66(3):542–51.

Kaasalainen S, Brazil K, Akhtar-Danesh N, Coker E, Ploeg J, Donald F, et al. The evaluation of an interdisciplinary pain protocol in long-term care. JAMDA. 2012;13:664e1–8.

Kaasalainen S, Ploeg J, Donald F, Coker E, Brazil K, Martin-Misener R, et al. Positioning clinical nurse specialists and nurse practitioners as change champions to implement a pain protocol in long-term care. Pain Manag Nurs. 2015;16(2):78–88.

Kaasalainen S, Wickson-Griffiths A, Akhtar-Danesh A, Brazil K, Donald F, Martin-Misener R, et al. The effectiveness of nurse practitioner-led pain management team in long-term care: a mixed methods study. Int J Nurs Stud. 2016;62:156–67.

Kee CC, Epps CD. Pain management practices of nurses caring for older adult patients with osteoarthritis. West J Nurs Res. 2001;23(2):195–210.

Long CO. Pain management education in long-term care: it can make a difference. Pain Manag Nurs. 2013;14(4):220–7.

Long CO, Morgan BMMM, Alonzo TR, Mitchell KM, Bonnell DK, Beardsley M. Improving pain management in long-term care: the "campaign against pain". J Hosp Palliat Nurs. 2010;12(3):148–55.

MacSorley R, White J, Conerly VH, Walker JT, Lofton S, Ragland G, et al. Pain assessment and management strategies for elderly patients. Home Healthc Nurse. 2014;32(5):272–85.

Muntinga ME, Jansen APD, Schellevis FG, Nijpels G. Expanding access to pain care for frail, old people in primary care: a cross-sectional study. BMC Nurs. 2016;15:26.

Musclow SL, Sawhney M, Watt-Watson J. The emerging role of advanced practice nursing in acute pain management throughout Canada. Clin Nurse Spec. 2002;16(2):62–7.

National Institutes of Health. Global health and aging [Report on the internet]. The Institute: 2011; [cited 18 Dec 2017]. p. 32. Available from http://www.who.int/ageing/publications/global_health.pdf.

Ontario Long-Term Care Association. This is long-term care 2016. [Report available on the internet]. 2016; [cited 18 Dec 2017] p. 16. Available from https://www.oltca.com/OLTCA/Documents/Reports/TILTC2016.pdf.

Park HR, Park E, Park JW. Barriers to chronic pain management in community-dwelling low-income older adults: home visiting-nurses' perspectives. Collegian. 2016;23:257–64.

RNAO. Assessment and management of pain in the elderly: a self-directed learning package for nurses in long-term care [Document available on the internet]. 2007; [cited 18 Dec 2017]. Available from http://rnao.ca/sites/rnao-ca/files/Assessment_and_Management_of_Pain_in_the_Elderly_-_Learning_Package_for_LTC.pdf.

RNAO. Assessment and management of pain (3rd ed.). [Document available on the internet]. 2013; [cited 18 Dec 2017]. Available from http://rnao.ca/bpg/guidelines/assessment-and-management-pain.

Royal College of Nurses. RCN Pain Knowledge and Skills Framework for the nursing team. (2015). [cited 18 Dec 2017]. Available from https://www.britishpainsociety.org/static/uploads/resources/files/RCN_KSF_2015.pdf.

Schofield P. Pain education and current curricula for older adults. Pain Med. 2012;13(supp 2):S51–6.

Stollee P, Hillier LM, Esbaugh J, Griffiths N, Borrie MJ. Examining the nurse practitioner role in long-term care: evaluation of a pilot project in Canada. J Gerontol Nurs. 2006;32(10):28–36.

Swafford KL, Miller LL, Herr K, Forcucci C, Kelly AML, Bakerjian D. Geriatric pain competencies and knowledge assessment for nurses in long-term care settings. Geriatr Nurs. 2014;35:423–7.

The Australian Pain Society [Internet]. 2017. [cited 18 Dec 2017]. Available from https://www.apsoc.org.au/.

The British Pain Society [Internet]. 2017. [cited 18 Dec 2017]. Available from https://www.britishpainsociety.org/.

The Canadian Pain Society [Internet]. 2017. [cited 18 Dec 2017]. Available from http://www.canadianpainsociety.ca/.

The University of Iowa [Internet]. Geriatricpain.org resources and tools for quality pain care. 2017. [cited 18 Dec 2017]. Available from https://geriatricpain.org/.

Tsai IP, Jeong SYM, Hunter S. Pain assessment and management for older patients with dementia in hospitals: an integrative literature review. Pain Manag Nurs. 2017;19(1):54–71.

Tse MYM, Ho SSK. Pain management for older persons living in nursing homes: a pilot study. Pain Manag Nurs. 2013;14(2):e10–21.

Wickson-Griffiths A, Kaasalainen S, Herr K. Interdisciplinary approaches to managing pain in older adults. Clin Geriatr Med. 2016;32:693–704.

Wiles JL, Leibing A, Guberman N, Reeve J, Allen RE. The meaning of "ageing in place" to older people. The Gerontologist. 2011;52(3):357–66. https://doi.org/10.1093/geront/gnr098.

Attitudes and Barriers to Pain Management in the Ageing Population

Paul A. Cameron, Rebecca Chandler, and Pat Schofield

Abstract
- There will be increased numbers of older adults in society in the next few decades.
- Older adults are more likely to have pain problems and other co-morbidities.
- Generally, pain is poorly managed in older adults, and this becomes worse when cognitive impairment exists.
- The impact of chronic pain on older adults will be greater than that of their younger counterparts in terms of social isolation.
- Attitudes and barriers to improved pain management exist in both the older adults themselves and their younger counterparts

The population is ageing; it is anticipated that the age distribution over 65 years will rise to 36% by 2050, and with the potential to live longer, it has been suggested that we will see the over 80 age group triple in numbers. With the frequency of pain being reported to be as high as 73% in community-dwelling older adults and increasing to 80% of those living in care homes, there is the potential for an ageing pain "time bomb". It is not just chronic pain either; studies demonstrate that acute pain

P. A. Cameron
Scottish Government, NHS Fife Pain Service, University of Dundee,
Dundee, UK

R. Chandler
Positive Ageing Research Institute, Anglia Ruskin University, Chelmsford, UK

P. Schofield (✉)
Department of Nursing, Anglia Ruskin University, Chelmsford, UK
e-mail: patricia.schofield@anglia.ac.uk

© Springer International Publishing AG, part of Springer Nature 2018
G. Pickering et al. (eds.), *Pain Management in Older Adults*, Perspectives in Nursing Management and Care for Older Adults, https://doi.org/10.1007/978-3-319-71694-7_9

is poorly managed in this group too (Desbiens et al. 1997). Sixty-seven percent of cancer deaths occur in those over the age of 65, and with cancer comes pain (D'Agostino et al. 1990). Other common non-malignant pain conditions seen in older people include osteoarthritis, postherpetic neuralgia, poststroke pain, and diabetic neuropathy.

The management of chronic pain within an older age group requires that distinctive needs be met, often based on age-related biological, physical, and social changes. As if this were not enough, cultural misconceptions regarding an older adult's perception of pain can be a more difficult barrier to challenge effectively. Therefore, in order to address attitudes of healthcare professionals in managing chronic pain in older adults, it is important to first understand how these professionals view the management needs of older adults with chronic pain.

The attitudes of healthcare professionals have impact on the management of those with chronic pain (Shaw and Lee 2010; Ryan et al. 2010), and these attitudes should be better understood in order to improve healthcare professionals' education at pre- and post-graduate level (Akesson et al. 2003; Leo et al. 2003). With these attitudes, we often see poor pain management as a result.

Furthermore, pain is common amongst older adults with dementia, with estimations indicating between 50 and 80% of this group experiencing regular pain (Corbett et al. 2012; Achterberg et al. 2013). Despite this, assessment and treatment of pain in this vulnerable population is frequently inadequate, with studies indicating older adults with dementia receive less pain relief than they require and subsequently experience negative physiological and psychological consequences (De Witt Jansen et al. 2017). The underlying reasons for such high prevalence figures and inadequate treatment represent the interplay of a number of barriers which preclude pain being recognised and treated appropriately.

There are many attitudinal barriers which exist both in healthcare and amongst the older population themselves. These are often described as misconceptions.

Some of the common misconceptions about chronic pain in the older population include:

It is a sign of personal weakness to acknowledge chronic pain.
Chronic pain is a punishment for past actions.
Chronic pain means death is near.
Chronic pain always indicates the presence of a serious disease.
Acknowledging pain will lead to a loss of independence.
Older people, especially the cognitively impaired, have a higher tolerance for pain.
Older people and the cognitively impaired cannot accurately self-report pain.
Residents in long-term care say they are in pain in order to get attention.
Older residents are likely to become addicted to pain medication.

Whilst we are aware that there are many barriers to effective pain management across the age spectrum and including older adults, for example, lack of knowledge, and lack of effective pain assessment tools. It seems that attitudes are a major factor which presents a barrier to effective pain management in the older population. Therefore, factors influencing barriers and attitudes will be discussed in more detail below.

A recent study by Cameron et al. (2015) asked a direct question regarding the need to have different management approaches for chronic pain in older people, but found that participants in their study did not see age to be an influencing factor in the choice of approaches. However, they also found that at over 75 years of age, access is harder than for younger adults for myriad reasons. Therefore, modification in management is required.

Previous studies have found similar patterns when measuring attitudes towards back pain[21]. When asked about their treatment orientation towards chronic low back pain, physiotherapy students were noted to hold different explicit and implicit attitudes, and these differences were found to influence behaviour and treatment approaches. This suggests that those who are involved in treating pain may not be explicitly aware of their own attitudes, or how it may change their behaviour when treating patients.

9.1   Mobility and the Fear of Mobility

Healthcare professionals often talk about aspects of mobility when considering pain in older adults—from suppositions as to how older adults would like to keep active to statements about the medical need to keep active. In interviews conducted, healthcare professionals talked of the importance of movement when considering pain management in older adults, although differences were noted in the extent to which they felt it important. Several studies commend the importance of movement in older adults, citing lower mortality rates and fewer hospital stays as a consequence (Carter et al. 2001; Morone and Greco 2007; Howe et al. 2007).

In a study by Cameron et al. (2015), a perceived fear of mobility is something healthcare professionals feel they experienced in their older patients. In many cases this was not actually expressed by patients, but an assumption by healthcare professionals, who correlate lack of movement to a fear of movement. Additionally, healthcare professionals themselves are fearful of causing damage to an older adult through their encouragement of movement. Despite evidence that movement, even in the presence of pain, is beneficial, often healthcare professionals are fearful of providing advice and information to increase activity in the older population, for fear of causing injury.

9.2   Psychology, Negative Thoughts, Coping, and Reinforcement

The influence of a therapist-patient relationship on treatment outcome has found that a positive relationship leads to a more positive treatment outcome (Hall et al. 2010). Trust, compassion, communication, competency, and privacy were all viewed as vital to cooperation with treatment (McKinstry et al. 2006). However, statements made by healthcare professionals have been found to indicate a tendency for pre-conceived ideas to influence treatment recommendation and expectation. Expressing a belief that older adults tend to cope with their pain suggests a pre-existing attitude that may predispose a clinician in failing to ask an older adult how they are coping. Coping with pain may require several forms of support. It is likely that those forms will remain unknown if not discussed with the patient.

Healthcare professionals have articulated ideas around an older adult's psychological strength and a decreased ability to cope or engage with strategies suggested. Often this was expressed in a way that would suggest that older adults are distinct in this need. Conversely, these statements are often negated by mention of experience and stoicism playing a part in an older adult's ability to self-manage. Whilst it is likely that an older adult's psychological strength does play a part in their ability to cope with pain, it is unlikely that this trait is unique to older adults.

9.3   Communication and Cognition

It is well recognised that older age carries an increased risk of cognitive decline, hearing loss, and visual impairment (Yorkston et al. 2010). However, not all older adults suffer from these difficulties, and many would not decrease an older adult's ability to understand concepts. Often communication adjustment is required when dealing with older adults. Communication with this population is not impossible, even when there is ongoing cognitive impairment. The issue is related to taking more time to explain and reinforce concepts to the older person and maybe even writing down instructions and explanations as an *aide memoire*.

Cognitive impairment is a concern amongst some clinicians who go so far as to doubt an older adult's account of their history of pain, even discounting further discussion with the older adult as it was unlikely to be useful. In studies examining methods of communication used with older adults, it was found that in those with cognitive impairment, rather than reducing attempts to communicate with them, it was more useful to change the approach to accommodate them. Taking extra time for communication, ensuring a friendly environment that was quiet and well lit, and understanding the patient's communication strengths and weaknesses were all suggested as strategies to use when communicating with those with cognitive impairment (Yorkston et al. 2010).

There is a lack of clarity amongst HCPs in relation to how pain is processed and experienced in older adults with dementia (Barry et al. 2012; Kenefick and Schulman-Green 2004). One study reported 80.5% of care home managers believe pain is experienced or processed differently in those with dementia compared to cognitively intact older adults (Barry et al. 2012). However conversely, Zwakhalen et al. (2007) found 72% of nurses and nursing assistants do not believe older adults with dementia experience any different or less pain. Similarly, Kenefick and Schulman-Green (2004) found nurses believe older adults with dementia do experience pain; however the difference is in their ability to understand and respond to sensory stimuli, such as pain-related questions. This lack of clarity amongst HCPs is not dissimilar from the current state of research in this area, which does not provide a clear image of the impact of neurological and biochemical disease changes on pain (Achterberg et al. 2013). It is therefore understandable how this ambiguity could translate into indecision in practice and unsuitable treatment choices (Achterberg et al. 2013).

In dementia, pain may be expressed through challenging or unusual behaviour (Achterberg et al. 2013), and untreated pain may contribute to behavioural and psychological symptoms of dementia (BPSD), depression, frailty, sleep disturbances, and reduced social activity (Griffioen et al. 2017; Flo et al. 2017). Together this can complicate the manifestation of pain; however research indicates nurses demonstrate a clear understanding of how pain might be communicated behaviourally (Kovach et al. 2000). It has been found that nurses are able to identify numerous relevant pain indicators, such as restlessness, grimacing, and behavioural changes. However, they do not feel confident in their knowledge of this, indicating assessing pain in dementia is a guessing game (Kovach et al. 2000). This lack of confidence might be reinforced by the attitude that behavioural manifestations of pain cannot be definitely identified from the symptoms of dementia (Kenefick and Schulman-Green 2004). The result of this uncertainty could be inappropriate use of psychotic medications in which pain is either ignored or mistreated (Kenefick and Schulman-Green 2004). Familiarity with a patient however is believed to mediate the uncertainty in identifying pain, enabling challenging or unusual behaviours to be recognised as expressions of pain rather than related to the disease symptoms (19).

9.4 Assessment of Pain in Adults with Dementia

Dementia-specific observational pain assessment tools (PATs) have been developed to assist in the identification of pain via observation of behaviours and verbalisations indicative of pain (see Chap. 3). Guidelines for the assessment and management of pain in older adults with cognitive impairment advocate the use of observational PATs to identify pain and to determine the efficacy of pain management given. However, research indicates healthcare staff and nurses do not use observational PATs for either purpose (Liu et al. 2011; Peisah et al. 2014; Barry et al. 2015). It has been found that nursing home staff believe observational PATs are too time-consuming, are inconvenient for routine use, lack standardisation, are difficult to interpret, are too generic, and are subjective (Liu et al. 2011). They do however believe they are useful to increase nursing staff's awareness of pain or for those inexperienced in dementia (Liu et al. 2011). Ultimately, the feeling amongst HCPs is that professional experience and judgement is more accurate and superior to formalised PATs (Kenefick and Schulman-Green 2004).

Interestingly, despite reporting non-use of observational PATs, studies have found that informal observational skills and knowledge is incorporated into daily practices (Liu et al. 2011). De Witt Jansen et al. (2017) found healthcare assistants engage in relationship-centred pain assessment during daily care exercises. Nursing assistants use their awareness of dementia residents' usual behaviours to identify when behavioural changes occur and identify possible causes of pain (De Witt Jansen et al. 2017).

In the early stages of dementia, self-report PATs can be used; these require an older adult with dementia to indicate the level or intensity of their pain based on numbers, words, or faces (Achterberg et al. 2013). Attitudes towards the use of self-report amongst HCPs vary between studies, perhaps reflecting the different degrees of dementia each group provide care for. Studies find that both nurses and nursing home managers (over 90%) do not believe older adults with dementia can provide an accurate self-report of pain or comprehend pain-related questions (Barry et al. 2012; Gilmore-Bykovskyi and Bowers 2013). It has further been found that older adults with dementia who do not present with the "correct" patient or pain characteristics, despite self-reporting pain, have their pharmacological pain management deferred (Gilmore-Bykovskyi and Bowers 2013). Older adults with severe dementia, no obvious injury, and a history of drug seeking and who have been a long-stay resident are reportedly perceived as least reliable to self-report their own pain (Gilmore-Bykovskyi and Bowers 2013). This suggests that attitudes towards dementia and what is characterised as the "correct" presentation of pain prevent effective pain management. In contrast to these other studies, Martin et al. (Martin et al. 2005) found a subset of nursing home staff who believed self-report from older adults with dementia could be accurately attained providing simple questions are used.

9.5   Physiology, Co-morbidities, and Signs of Ageing

Multiple pathologies in any one individual are not a phenomenon reserved specifically for older adults. Nevertheless there are some co-morbidities that are more common in older adults and cannot be ignored. Eight co-morbidities have been highlighted as commonly affecting older adults (Harris and Guzzo 2013): deep vein thrombosis (DVT), functional loss, immobility, delirium, post-operative cognitive dysfunction, urinary tract infection (UTI), falls, and frailty. Furthermore, Cameron et al. (2015) noted that sensitivity to medication was a common concern for healthcare professionals. Professionals were often concerned with causing iatrogenic harm, as a consequence of changes in an older adult's ability to physiologically manage their medication. There was also some concern that the clinician may not necessarily have the specialised knowledge required to manage these issues.

9.6   Pharmacological Interventions

Pharmacokinetic changes do occur in older adults. However, there is no agreement as to the point that this occurs, nor is it the same in each individual. Some older adults may cope with medication in the same manner as some younger counterparts; equally some may cope less well. It is likely that the oldest-old, commonly considered as above 85 (AgeUK 2013), will present with more pharmacokinetic age-related changes, but other older adults may not. However, attitudes that consider age when considering medicine management may be appropriate, if treatment is given on an individual basis. To illustrate this point, recent UK guidelines on the management of pain in older adults (Schofield 2013) do not exclude medication for use with older adults and suggest using stronger opioids over weaker opioids in some instances to reduce commonly seen side-effects when using weaker opioids (Schofield 2013).

Knowledge and attitudes towards the use of pharmacological interventions in older adults with dementia vary dependent on the form of pharmacology referred to. In relation to opioid analgesics, both nurses and nursing home managers express uncertainty about the safety and risks, including tolerance and addiction (Barry et al. 2012; Burns and McIlfatrick 2015; Kaasalainen et al. 2007). Nurses believe they should only be used as a last resort in dementia, particularly as certainty of the presence of pain cannot be established (Kaasalainen et al. 2007). However, in the context of palliative care, opioid analgesics and side-effects are considered to be acceptable for the relief of the patient (Brorson et al. 2013; De Witt Jansen et al. 2017). In addition, where oral administration is precluded, opioid analgesics provide alternative methods of administration, such as injections; however these are perceived to add additional distress and discomfort to palliative dementia patients (De Witt Jansen et al. 2017).

More positive attitudes are expressed towards the use of non-steroidal anti-inflammatory drugs (NSAIDs) and paracetamol with nursing home managers, nurses, and healthcare assistants reacting positively towards their use in dementia (Barry et al. 2012; Kovach et al. 2000). The risks of NSAIDs and paracetamol are believed to outweigh the costs, particularly in contrast to narcotic medications (Kovach et al. 2000). All groups endorsed a step-wise approach as safest and most effective (Barry et al. 2012; Kovach et al. 2000).

In contrast to this, Zwakhalen et al. (2007) found nursing staff were unsure about pain medications and concerned about side-effects, dosage, and addiction, over and above the relief of pain. Another area of confusion is medicating older adults with dementia, only around 60% of nursing home managers recognise pain should be medicated the same as in the cognitively intact (Barry et al. 2012). Such deficits in understanding may explain why older adults with dementia receive significantly less pain relief than other older adults despite suffering comparable pain conditions (Barry et al. 2012; De Witt Jansen et al. 2017).

9.7   Non-pharmacological Pain Management

UK guidelines for the management of pain in older adults do suggest some non-pharmacological approaches to pain management (e.g. The British Geriatrics Society 2013); however these methods are yet to be evidenced fully in dementia. Knowledge of non-pharmacological methods is limited amongst healthcare staff; however findings do indicate nursing staff and nurses perceive it to be a useful compliment to pharmacological methods, particularly during palliative care (Brorson et al. 2013; Martin et al. 2005). Nurses indicate these methods can be individualised to the patient, highlighting the use of music and hand-holding to relieve anxiety and distress (Martin et al. 2005).

9.8   Attitudes of Older Adults Themselves

A number of reasons have been highlighted earlier which seek to explain why pain is poorly managed in older adults compared to their younger counterparts. There is a lack of evidence regarding acceptable treatment for older adults (Gibson 2006) as trials tend to focus upon younger adults, and it is acknowledged that older adults are under-represented in pain clinics and pain management programmes (Kee et al. 1998). Other reasons cited include the fact that pain is assumed to be part of ageing, older adults assume that healthcare professionals will "know" when they are in pain, and of course, with increased age comes the increased likelihood of co-morbidities which can complicate diagnosis and cause unpleasant interactions with medications thus affecting concordance. With increasing age and the potential vulnerability comes the risk of cognitive impairment which can make diagnosis more difficult.

A recent qualitative study sought to identify some of the barriers to reporting pain held by residents themselves living in a number of care homes within one district (Schofield 2013). A series of semi-structured interviews were conducted with residents who were mildly/moderate cognitively impaired. The interviews identified a number of key themes as follows:

1. A reluctance to report pain/acceptance that pain is normal and low expectations of help from medical interventions. Many residents when interviewed were in pain, but when asked why they had not reported the pain to the staff, they commented that there was no need to, as there was probably nothing that anyone could do.
2. Fear of chemical/pharmacological interventions. Many of the residents commented that they were fearful of using pharmacological interventions, and they would prefer to manage without, or that nothing seemed to help.
3. Age-related perceptions of pain. Not only were the older age group (>80) reluctant to take analgesics, but they were also reluctant to actually admit that they had pain. The residents under 75 years were more willing to voice their pain, and consequently to take analgesic drugs.

9.9   Need for Training

Many of the studies cited also reported the training received in each of their samples, between 60.4 and 90% had not received any training relating to pain or dementia (Peisah et al. 2014; Barry et al. 2015; Gibson 2006). Given this large deficit in training, it is not surprising that the HCP groups discussed the lack of knowledge and have negative attitudes in some areas. It is evident from some of the practices reported above, such as non-use of PAT, pain management protocols and guidelines are not referred to. This is reinforced by findings that guidelines and protocols are only used in 60% of instances when available (Barry et al. 2015; Martin et al. 2005). Despite this all, HCP groups across studies recognised pain was being poorly managed in older adults with dementia, expressing a deep concern and empathy for this vulnerable group (Barry et al. 2015; Kaasalainen et al. 2007; Martin et al. 2005). They too recognised their need for further education, communicating a desire to receive relevant education (Barry et al. 2015; Martin et al. 2005).

Conclusion

Older adults are increasing within our society. It is well documented that they have poor pain management, and this is attributed to barriers and attitudes which influence beliefs amongst healthcare professionals and the older population themselves. In order to address these issues, we need to educate all staff to understand that poor pain management is unacceptable, and we need to change the attitudes of older adults themselves to help them understand that they can complain and they do have a "right" to effective pain management. We know that pain severity is strongly correlated with quality of life, and severity of pain increases with increasing age. If we are to improve the pain in this population, this chapter shows that we need to change the attitudes which pervade around this issue.

References

Achterberg WP, Pieper MJ, van Dalen-Kok AH, de Waal MWM, Husebo BS, Lautenbacher S, et al. Pain management in patients with dementia. Clin Interv Aging. 2013;8:1471–82. https://doi.org/10.2147/CIA.S36739.

AgeUK. Oldest old in the United Kingdom – a Factsheet for Professionals. 2013. http://www.ageuk.org.uk/Documents/EN-GB/For-professionals/Research/Oldest%20Old%20in%20the%20UK%20fact%20sheet%20(8%203%2013).doc.

Akesson K, Dreinhofer KE, Woolf AD. Improved education in musculoskeletal conditions is necessary for all doctors. Bull World Health Organ. 2003;81(9):677–83.

Barry HE, Parson C, Passmore PA, Hughes CM. An exploration of nursing home managers' knowledge of and attitudes towards the management of pain in residents with dementia. Int J Geriatr Psychiatry. 2012;27:1258–66. https://doi.org/10.1002/gps.3770.

Barry HE, Parson C, Passmore PA, Hughes CM. Pain in care home residents with dementia: an exploration of frequency, prescribing and relatives' perspectives. Int J Geriatr Psychiatry. 2015;30:55–63. https://doi.org/10.1002/gps.4111.

Brorson H, Plymoth H, Ãrmon K, Bolmsj ÃI. Pain relief at the end of life: nurses' experiences regarding end-of-life pain relief in patients with dementia. Pain Manag Nurs. 2013;15:315–23. https://doi.org/10.1016/j.pmn.2012.10.005.

Burns M, McIlfatrick S. Nurses' knowledge and attitudes towards pain assessment for people with dementia in a nursing home setting. Int J Palliat Nurs. 2015;21:479–87. https://doi.org/10.12968/ijpn.2015.21.10.479.

Cameron PA, Smith BH, Schofield PA. Healthcare professionals' accounts of chronic pain management for older adults. J Pain Rehabil. 2015;38:17–27.

Carter ND, Kannus P, Khan K. Exercise in the prevention of falls in older people. Sports Med. 2001;31(6):427–38.

Corbett A, Husebo B, Malcangio M, Staniland A, Cohen-Mansfield J, Aarsland D, et al. Assessment and treatment of pain in people with dementia. Nat Rev Neurol. 2012;8:264–74. https://doi.org/10.1038/nrneurol.2012.53.

D'Agostino NS, Gray G, Scanlon C. J Gerontol Nurs. 1990;16:12–5.

De Witt Jansen B, Brazil K, Passmore P, Buchanan H, Maxwell D, Mcllfactrick SJ, et al. Exploring healthcare assistants' role and experience in pain assessment and management for people with advanced dementia towards the end of life: a qualitative study. BMC Palliat Care. 2017;16:1–11. https://doi.org/10.1186/s12904-017-0184-1.

Desbiens NA, Mueller-Rizner N, Connors AF. J Am Geriatr Soc. 1997;45:1167–72.

Flo E, Bjorvatn B, Corbett A, Pallesen S, Husebo BS. Joint occurrence of pain and sleep disturbances in people with dementia. Curr Alzheimer Res. 2017;14:538–45. https://doi.org/10.2174/1567205013666160602234932.

Gibson SJ. Pain Clin Updates. 2006;14:1–4.

Gilmore-Bykovskyi AL, Bowers BJ. Understanding nurses' decision to treat pain in nursing home residents with dementia. Res Gerontol Nurs. 2013;6:127–38. https://doi.org/10.3928/19404921-20130110-02.

Griffioen C, Willems EG, Husebo BS, Achterberg WP. Prevalence of the use of opioids for treatment of pain in persons with a cognitive impairment compared with cognitively intact persons: a systematic review. Curr Alzheimer Res. 2017;14:512–22. https://doi.org/10.2174/1567205013666160629080735.

Hall AM, Ferreira PH, Maher CG, Latimer J, Ferreira ML. The influence of the therapist-patient relationship on treatment outcome on physical rehabilitation: a systematic review. Phys Ther. 2010;90(8):1099–110.

Harris AM, Guzzo TJ. Chapter 6. Complications particular to the elderly. In: Primer of geriatric urology. New York: Springer; 2013.

Howe TE, Rochester L, Jackson A, Banks PMH, Blair VA. Exercise for improving balance in older people. In: Cochrane database of systematic reviews, vol. 4. New Jersey: Wiley; 2007.

Kaasalainen S, et al. Pain management decision-making among long-term care physicians and nurses. West J Nurs Res. 2007;29:561–80.

Kee WG, Middaugh SJ, Redpath S, et al. Age as a factor in admission to chronic pain rehabilitation. Clin J Pain. 1998;14:121–8.

Kenefick A, Schulman-Green D. Caring for cognitively impaired nursing home residents with pain. IJHC. 2004;8:32–40.

Kovach CR, Griffie J, Muchka S, Noonan PE, Weissman DE. Nurses' perceptions of pain assessment and treatment in the cognitively impaired elderly. It's not a guessing game. Clin Nurse Spec. 2000;14:215–20.

Leo R, Pristach C, Streltzer J. Incorporating pain management training into the psychiatry residency programme. Acad Psychiatry. 2003;27(1):1–11.

Liu J, Briggs M, Closs J. Acceptability of Pain Behaviour Observational Methods (PBOMs) for use by nursing home staff. J Clin Nurs. 2011;20:2071–3. https://doi.org/10.1111/j.1365-2702.2010.03671.x.

Martin R, Williams J, Hadjistavropoulos T, Hadjistavropoulos H, MacLean M. A qualitative investigation of 'seniors and caregivers' views on pain assessment and management. Can J Nurs Res. 2005;37:142–64.

McKinstry B, Ashcroft RE, Car J, Freeman GK, Sheikh A. Interventions for improving patients' trust in doctors and groups of doctors. Cochrane Libr. 2006;3:CD004134.

Morone NE, Greco CM. Mind-body interventions for older adults: a structured review. Pain Med. 2007;8(4):359–75.

Peisah C, Weaver J, Wong L, Strukovski J. Silent and suffering: a pilot study exploring gaps between theory and practice in pain management for people with severe dementia in residential aged care facilities. Clin Interv Aging. 2014;9:1767–74. https://doi.org/10.2147/CIA.S64598.

Ryan C, Murphy D, Clark M, Lee A. The effect of a physiotherapy education compared with a non-healthcare education on the attitudes and beliefs of students towards functioning in individuals with back pain. An observational, cross-sectional study. Physiotherapy. 2010;96:144–50.

Schofield P. Guidance on the management of pain in older people. Age Ageing. 2013;42 (Supp 1):i1–i57.

The British Geriatric Society. Guidance for the management of pain in older adults. Guidelines 1st October. The British Geriatric Society. London, UK; 2013.

Shaw S, Lee A. Student nurses misconceptions of adults with chronic nonmalignant pain. Pain Manag Nurs. 2010;11(1):2–14.

Yorkston KM, Bourgeois MS, Baylor CR. Communication and aging. Phys Med Rehabil Clin Neurol Am. 2010;21(2):309–19.

Zwakhalen SM, Hamers JP, Penijenburg RH, Berger MP. Nursing staff knowledge and beliefs about pain in elderly nursing home residents. Pain Res Manag. 2007;12:177–84.

Translating Knowledge to Improve Pain Management Practices for Older Adults

10

Esther Coker and Sharon Kaasalainen

Abstract

Translation of pain management evidence into practice is slow, and therefore pain in older adults continues to be under-recognized and under-treated. Several barriers to pain management in older adults have been identified, and they may be addressed through implementation science—the study of methods to promote integration of research findings into policy and practice. Successful knowledge translation relies on the use of a conceptual framework to guide the development, implementation, and sustainability of evidence-based pain management strategies. The Knowledge to Action and Promoting Action on Research Implementation in Health Services frameworks lend themselves to this purpose.

Knowledge translation involves behaviour change, especially around nurses' decision-making. Some of the knowledge translation interventions applied to pain management are educational meetings, audit and feedback, reminders, opinion leaders and change champions, educational outreach, and appreciative inquiry. Tailoring interventions to address barriers can serve to support implementation of pain guideline recommendations. Determinants of guideline uptake are outlined in this chapter along with factors impacting the sustainability of use of guidelines. Leadership involvement; credible evidence; staff buy-in and education; experiencing small, successive "wins"; and monitoring and feedback contribute to successful implementation of pain management clinical practice guidelines.

E. Coker (✉)
Hamilton Health Sciences, Hamilton, ON, Canada

McMaster University School of Nursing, Hamilton, ON, Canada
e-mail: coker@hhsc.ca; cokerme@mcmaster.ca

S. Kaasalainen
McMaster University School of Nursing, Hamilton, ON, Canada
e-mail: kaasal@mcmaster.ca

© Springer International Publishing AG, part of Springer Nature 2018
G. Pickering et al. (eds.), *Pain Management in Older Adults*, Perspectives in Nursing Management and Care for Older Adults, https://doi.org/10.1007/978-3-319-71694-7_10

121

10.1 Introduction

Managing pain in older people is challenging because they tend to be frail, they have more comorbidities, often have complex medication regimes associated with other diseases, and are more susceptible to conditions such as dementia that can confound pain assessment (Savvas et al. 2015). Older people are also prone to a range of pain conditions including osteoarthritis and neuropathic pain syndromes and can at times also require postoperative pain management. Pain management practices comprise (a) screening for pain, (b) timely and appropriate comprehensive pain assessment for both patients whose screen reveals the presence of pain and for those who cannot self-report, (c) establishing a comprehensive treatment plan, (d) pharmacologic and non-pharmacologic interventions for pain, and (e) continuous evaluation of those treatments and possible side effects.

While internationally there are a number of guidelines and recommendations on the management of pain in older adults, translation of evidence into practice is slow, and under-recognition and under-treatment of pain continue (Douglas et al. 2016; Schofield et al. 2012). This phenomenon is not unique to the older adult population—it is observed in the field of paediatric pain management as well (Foster 2013; Scott-Findlay and Estabrooks 2006; Stevens 2009). In fact, according to Grimshaw and colleagues, this failure to translate research into policy and practice is one of the most consistent findings in clinical and health services research (Grimshaw et al. 2012). The purpose of this chapter is to explore strategies to promote successful implementation of pain management practices with older adults.

10.2 Barriers to Pain Management

In Chap. 9 a number of barriers to optimal pain management were outlined. An integrative review of the literature on pain management revealed barriers related to patient characteristics, professional knowledge and education, and the setting (Ortiz et al. 2014). Individual patient barriers included negative patient attitudes and beliefs, lack of patient involvement, inability to communicate pain due to cognition or language barriers, under-reporting pain (sometimes because of an inadequate pain tool), and attitudes toward analgesics. Barriers at the professional level included inadequate education, attitudes and beliefs (e.g. overly conservative pain management), lack of interprofessional collaboration, inability to access pain experts, inconsistent approaches, lack of documentation, lack of confidence, and misinformed decision-making. Organizational barriers included workplace dynamics, workplace culture and practice, demanding workloads and lack of time, lack of standardized pain assessment and documentation tools, inadequate pain protocols, and scope of practice (e.g. inability to prescribe resulting in delays) (Ortiz et al. 2014). Other barriers to optimal pain management reported in the literature include staff and leadership turnover, state of science around pain in older adults, and traditional clinical behaviours or previous practices of nurses (Kaasalainen et al. 2010; Ersek et al. 2016; Carlson 2010). The barriers to effective pain management practices identified in the literature may inform implementation science research.

10.3   Implementation Science

Implementation science is the study of methods to promote the integration of research findings and evidence into health-care policy and practice. The purpose of implementation science research is to address barriers (e.g. social, behavioural, economic, management) to effective implementation of research findings, test new approaches, and determine the relationship between the intervention and its impact (National Information Center on Health Services Research and Health Care Technology (NICHSR) 2017). Understanding the behaviour of nurses and other stakeholders is an important factor in the sustainable uptake, adoption, and implementation of evidence-based interventions such as pain management practices.

Knowledge translation (KT) is defined as a dynamic and iterative process to improve health, provide more effective health services and products, and strengthen the health-care system (Graham et al. 2006). The four elements of knowledge translation are (a) synthesis, (b) dissemination, (c) exchange, and (d) ethically sound application of knowledge (Canadian Institutes of Health Research 2016).

Synthesis involves integrating the research findings of individual research studies on pain assessment and management within the larger body of knowledge on the topic. It could take the form of a systematic review of the literature, results from a consensus conference or expert panel, or a synthesis of qualitative or quantitative results. Narrative syntheses, meta-analyses, meta-syntheses, and practice guidelines are all forms of synthesis (Canadian Institutes of Health Research 2016).

Dissemination is the purposeful distribution of pain management information and materials to nurses. The intent is to spread information and the associated evidence-based interventions. Dissemination addresses how pain management information is created, packaged, transmitted, and interpreted among stakeholders (National Information Center on Health Services Research and Health Care Technology (NICHSR) 2017).

Knowledge exchange is the collaborative problem-solving that takes place between pain management researchers and nurse decision-makers. Effective knowledge exchange results in mutual learning through the process of planning, producing, disseminating, and applying existing or new research in decision-making (Canadian Foundation for Healthcare Improvement 2017).

Application is the iterative process by which knowledge about pain management is put into practice (Canadian Institutes of Health Research 2016). Evaluation and monitoring of KT initiatives, processes, and activities are key components of the KT process.

10.4   The Need for Frameworks in Knowledge Translation

Until recently, implementation science had a limited theoretical basis which made it difficult to determine how and why implementation succeeds or fails and what strategies could be used to achieve success (Nilsen 2015; Rycroft-Malone et al. 2013). There is now a generally accepted need to utilize conceptual frameworks that can describe and measure the components of a successful knowledge translation process.

A narrative review conducted by Nilsen (2015) revealed five categories of theories, models and frameworks used in implementation science: (a) process models, including the Knowledge to Action framework by Graham et al. (2006), meant to describe and guide the process of translating research into practice; (b) determinant frameworks, including the Promoting Action on Research Implementation in Health Services (PARIHS) framework by Rycroft-Malone et al. (2013), which explain how barriers and enablers influence implementation outcomes; (c) classic theories, including the Diffusion of Innovations by Rogers (2003), which originate from other fields and explain aspects of implementation; (d) implementation theories; and (e) evaluation frameworks.

Milat and Li (2017) conducted a review of frameworks for translating research evidence into policy and practice. They identified 41 frameworks and models that have their origins in different fields, i.e. implementation science, basic science, medical science, health services research, and public health. They suggested that two models in particular lend themselves to practical application in the health services research field: the Knowledge to Action framework (Graham et al. 2006) and the PARIHS framework (Rycroft-Malone et al. 2013). The two models complement each other and can be used in the translation of knowledge in pain management. Both models are described in turn.

10.4.1 Knowledge to Action

Briefly, the Knowledge to Action framework comprises two components. The first is a knowledge creation "funnel" in which knowledge becomes more and more refined from knowledge inquiry, through knowledge synthesis, to the creation of knowledge tools. There is also an action cycle with seven phases that is influenced by the knowledge funnel. The elements of the cycle can occur simultaneously or sequentially and include (a) problem identification and review of select knowledge, (b) adaptation of knowledge to the context, (c) assessment of barriers to knowledge use, (d) implementation of tailored interventions, (e) monitoring knowledge use, (f) evaluation of outcomes, and (g) sustaining knowledge use (Graham et al. 2006).

10.4.2 PARIHS

The Promoting Action on Research Implementation in Health Services (PARIHS) framework considers three core elements, i.e. evidence, context, and facilitation, which are dynamic and interrelated. Essentially, successful implementation relies on interactions among: (1) evidence that is robust and meaningful to nurses and may be drawn from research, clinical experience, patients and families, and local context and environment; (2) a context (e.g. environment, decision-making processes, power and authority, leadership, culture, evaluation, and measurement) that is receptive; and (3) implementation processes that are appropriately facilitated (Rycroft-Malone et al. 2013; Brown and McCormack 2005). Each of the core elements of the PARIHS framework will be considered in turn.

10.5 Evidence

10.5.1 First and Second Generation Knowledge

The knowledge creation component of the Knowledge to Action cycle consists of three phases (Graham et al. 2006). Knowledge inquiry represents unrefined first-generation knowledge—hundreds of primary studies on pain management. Second-generation knowledge represents a synthesis of those studies. Examples would include the systematic review conducted by Zwakhalen and colleagues of pain assessment tools for use with patients with severe dementia (Zwakhalen et al. 2006) and the position statement by Herr and colleagues on pain assessment in patients unable to self-report (Herr et al. 2011). User-friendly synopses such as practice guidelines, algorithms, and other tools represent third-generation knowledge.

10.5.2 Third-Generation Knowledge

Clinical practice guidelines (CPGs), or best practice guidelines (BPGs) as they are also known, are designed to move the best available pain evidence into daily practice while standardizing practices and contributing to consistent care delivery by nurses. Examples include guidelines published by the American Medical Directors Association (2012), the Hartford Institute for Geriatric Nursing (Horgas et al. 2012), Australian Pain Society (2005), and the American Geriatrics Society (American Geriatrics Society Panel on Persistent Pain in Older Persons 2002). However, despite health-care organizations expending considerable effort on developing and adopting CPGs, there is still a large gap between what nurses know and what they actually do (Saunders 2015). Although such guidelines have contributed to advances in translating research into practice through a set of recommendations that guide clinical decision-making at the point of care, it is still not clear how to encourage their uptake into practice (Saunders 2015). The inconsistent implementation may be due in part to their not being in usable form for clinical practice—the summarized and synthesized evidence needs to be translated and packaged concisely in a form that has been adapted to the setting in which it will be used.

Saunders (2015) proposed that translation and packaging can be accomplished by creating pain management nursing (PMN) care bundles. Care bundles are sets of evidence-based practices that when implemented together in a reliable way will improve patient outcomes. They typically comprise three to five core interventions. A completely administered care bundle is documented as such, and compliance carefully monitored.

A large university hospital system in Finland used a care bundle approach to improve the uptake of CPGs on post-procedural pain management. Some of the strategies for successful implementation included translating the CPG into six actionable core nursing interventions, embedding the bundle into electronic documentation in the health record which also served as an audit tool, pilot testing and revising accordingly, training and identifying superusers, and creating a working group to oversee the project which continues to meet regularly to evaluate and communicate adherence. Preliminary results of the implementation of the care bundle were positive, and plans were made to spread it to other services (Saunders 2015). In contrast, an attempt by Ersek and colleagues to embed guidelines into algorithms did not change pain practice and outcomes in long-term care. Implementation barriers included staff and management turnover, attitudes, lack of readiness for change, and unwieldy processes (Ersek et al. 2016).

Published clinical practice guidelines have been used in some studies as a standard to evaluate current practices and direct change (Savvas et al. 2015; Song et al. 2015). Guidelines are frequently made into a user-friendly format, often a checklist. Kaasalainen and colleagues successfully implemented a pain protocol in long-term care that was based on best practice guidelines and implemented using a combination of outreach visits, a pain team, reminders, change champions, and audit and feedback (Kaasalainen et al. 2012). Using on-site champions and using a pain team were considered keys to success.

10.6 Context

10.6.1 Decision-Making

Knowledge translation involves behaviour change among nurses working in healthcare organizations. Behaviour change will ideally be based on nurses' ability to influence pain management decision-making rather than through a purely protocol-driven process (Scott-Findlay and Estabrooks 2006). According to Scott-Findlay and Estabrooks (2006), nurses' decision-making around pain management is influenced, sometimes in competing ways, by many stakeholders such as managers, peers, students, patients, and families. In knowledge translation, influences beyond the knowledge of research findings alone must be considered—personal preferences, professional group norms, and the values of the setting in which the decisions related to pain management are made. It is not a simple matter of filling a knowledge or research gap.

Scott-Findlay and Estabrooks (2006) explained that using research in practice requires behaviour change—especially behaviour change around decision-making which is complex, though possible. They suggested, based on their knowledge translation work in paediatric pain management, that developing strategies to weave research into peer-to-peer interactions, in which nurses naturally prefer to engage for knowledge and problem-solving, may be successful (Scott-Findlay and Estabrooks 2006; Estabrooks et al. 2005). This would mean involving respected and trusted colleagues to help give pain management research findings a bigger role in decision-making.

10.6.2 Leadership

In a multiple case study, Etheridge et al. (2014) studied the implementation of four best practice innovations in long-term care—two successful and two unsuccessful—to understand how leaders use a participative rather than authoritarian approach to "make things happen", "help things happen", and "let things happen" (Greenhalgh et al. 2004). Their findings, which could be applied to the implementation of a pain management programme, were related to the successful implementation of a restraint reduction and constipation prevention programme and the not-so-successful implementation of a continence promotion and falls prevention programme. The "make things happen" approach influences the process of change in a planned and orderly scientific way, and in the successful cases, this steadfast commitment to quality was demonstrated to staff. "Help things happen" involves enabling, negotiating, and influencing through social or technical means, and in the successful cases, these types of motivational resources were offered to staff. In "let things happen", the change process is influenced by unplanned and unpredictable emerging process. In the successful cases, this allowed for creativity among staff, tailoring the programme to the setting and encouraging engagement. Successful implementation had these elements in common: the change process was initiated at the unit level by staff who had a strong desire for change, they received an appropriate amount of support from the manager, and their early small successes led to sustained engagement. The following were seen to underlie unsuccessful implementation: the initiative was one of many competing projects; staff opinions were not sought so buy-in did not occur; there was no reliance on staff knowledge and skills at the outset; there was no built-in measurement or dissemination of outcomes as the project progressed, and no oversight of implementation (Etheridge et al. 2014).

Fleiszer et al. (2016) conducted a qualitative case study of the strategies used by unit-based leaders to sustain BPG implementation. They studied four units in an acute care hospital system where three BPGs had been implemented with varying degrees of programme sustainability. On units where BPGs were sustained, two particular strategies had been used by leaders. They (a) preserved the BPG as a unit priority despite competing priorities, and (b) they reinforced the BPG recommendations as practice standards. Six specific activities had a positive influence on BPG sustainability. First, the leadership team emphasized the rationale behind the practice changes and extended the period of time for implementation to be sure that changes were fully embedded into practice. Second, they featured the BPG recommendations in unit orientation and print materials for new staff, offered regular education for staff, and held additional education session to address slippage in practice. Third, they used verbal reminders and a visual reminder system on their patient census board using colour-coded magnets. Another strategy involved leaders being present to facilitate discussion during shift handover where nurses learned from each other. Evaluating performance through audit and feedback was another strategy and served to ensure continued improvement through locally collected data to supplement hospital system-generated data. Lastly, leaders tried to sustain best practices by nesting them within other initiatives—existing or new—rather than trying to manage many separate projects.

Jeffs et al. (2016) also studied the role of the unit manager, specifically in engaging staff in quality improvement efforts. The first theme that emerged was balancing having a visible presence with enabling staff through conversations, for example, to engage in and take the lead on their QI initiatives. The second theme was related to supporting flexible schedules so staff had enough time to manage Quality

Improvement (QI) work in light of their clinical work as busy clinical environments can prevent clinicians from being able to fully commit to QI.

10.7 Facilitation

As yet, there is inadequate evidence in the nursing literature to guide the development of strategies that will improve nurses' ability to use pain research in practice or to change their decision-making behaviours in the area of pain management. Because high-quality systematic reviews of pain management guideline implementation strategies do not exist, the choice of interventions has not had a theoretical foundation. However, a few strategies for knowledge translation in pain management have been reported and have been used alone or in combination. These will be examined under some of the knowledge translation interventions identified through systematic reviews conducted by the Cochrane Effective Practice and Organization of Care (EPOC) group (2015) and reported by Swafford et al. (2009) and Yost et al. (2014).

10.7.1 Implementation of a Framework

The implementation of a systematic process improvement framework such as "Plan, Do, Study, Act" was reported in two quality improvement studies on pain management practices. Typically current practices were evaluated and an action plan with measurable goals followed (Swafford et al. 2009).

10.7.2 Educational Meetings

Nurses may participate in conferences, in-service education offerings, or workshops. Drake and Williams (2017) conducted a systematic review of the effects of nursing education interventions on clinical outcomes of acute pain management in hospitals. The timing of the review commenced where a high-quality review by Twycross (2002) left off. They suggested that behaviour change techniques applied to nursing education in acute pain management may impact clinical outcomes. They also suggested that including components of behaviour change such as emotion, intrinsic motivation, professional identity, and the meaning for nurses of performing the specific tasks involved in the intervention could enrich future nursing pain management interventions more than merely providing information and skills training. For example, heightening empathy for the pain experience of older adults with dementia would be an example of targeting emotion to change behaviour. Twelve eligible studies contributed to the findings. In general, the frequency of appropriate documentation improved significantly, and some studies showed an increase in comprehensiveness of documentation. Patient pain scores did not necessarily decrease, nor did overall patient satisfaction with pain management increase as a result of education and training.

The majority of studies used a variety of didactic and interactive methods including role play or vignettes, group discussion, performance feedback, and extra ongoing support, and those interventions were seen to cover off many of the domains involved in health-care behaviour change (Michie et al. 2005). The domains targeted by educational interventions included (a) knowledge; (b) skills; (c) professional role identity; (d) beliefs about capability; (e) beliefs about consequences; (f) motivation and goals; (g) memory, attention, and decision-making; (h) environmental resources; (i) social influences; (j) emotion; (k) behavioural regulation; and (l) nature of the behaviours (Drake and Williams 2017; Michie et al. 2005).

10.7.3 Audit and Feedback

Audit and feedback is meant to change nurses' behaviour by summarizing clinical performance over a period of time through a review of health records or through observations. The feedback and action planning is based on the audit findings (Grimshaw et al. 2012). In some studies in Drake and Williams' review (2017), data were collected regularly and adjustments to original action plans made based on feedback (Swafford et al. 2009). In a study of unrelieved pain in postoperative patients, nurses perceived their pain management practices as being adequate, and since there was no impetus to change, this was seen as a potential deterrent to adopting evidence-based practices related to pain management (Carlson 2010). In such cases, audit and feedback of current performance can help stimulate behaviour change (Grimshaw et al. 2012).

10.7.4 Reminders

Reminders may be verbal, written, or computerized and serve to prompt the nurse to adhere to pain management guidelines. Douglas and colleagues introduced a pain identification tool that provided a structured approach to pain assessment and provided the tool in a pain resource pack which was provided in combination with workshops and small group activities. The combination of interventions was only partially effective at improving outcomes though staff found the tool to have clinical utility (Douglas et al. 2016). Nurses can be prompted to document pain assessments and interventions via structured electronic documentation systems (Song et al. 2015). Embedding pain assessment tools, timing reminders, and pain reassessment reminders following administration of medications can all serve as prompts.

10.7.5 Opinion Leaders and Change Champions

Local opinion leaders are educationally influential colleagues who are able to influence knowledge, attitudes, social norms, and behaviours regularly. Opinion leaders earn their status as informal leaders among their peer group and are generally exposed to external communication, and they themselves are innovative and accessible (Grimshaw et al. 2012).

In a study where an evidence-based pain protocol was introduced in long-term care, clinical nurse specialists and nurse practitioners were positioned as change champions—those who support and drive and innovation through. Those advanced practice nurses in turn used a combination of other knowledge translation interventions including educational outreach, reminders, and chart audit and feedback (Kaasalainen et al. 2015). In a study of the sources of practice knowledge among nurses, nurses were less likely to consult advanced practice nurses than they were to consult other nurses with whom they work (Estabrooks et al. 2005). This may have implications for ensuring active knowledge exchange with informal nursing leaders.

10.7.6 Educational Outreach

Educational outreach involves a trained person meeting with nurses in their setting in an effort to change practice (Grimshaw et al. 2012). In the pain management literature, this often takes the form of a pain team.

Feldman et al. (2016) described a pain team comprising three palliative care physicians who provided pain and palliative care consultations throughout a large complex care hospital also supported a unit caring for older patients with acute medical illnesses. The team on the acute unit had not felt empowered to make decisions about pain management, so the pain team members increased their presence by attending daily rounds for 6 months during a pilot project. The immersion of the pain team into the social network of the interprofessional acute care team increased the confidence of the latter. The pain team's role became that of collaboration rather than consultation by building positive and trusting relationships.

The majority of the quality improvement studies on process improvement of pain care in long-term care included in a literature synthesis by Swafford et al. (2009) reported having assembled a facility-based pain team to oversee the planning and implementation of process changes related to pain assessment and management. Pain champions were appointed at five residential aged care facilities that were aiming to improve compliance with pain management standards. The champions received additional training and were often members of the pain team (Savvas et al. 2015).

10.7.7 Appreciative Inquiry

Kavanagh et al. (2008) examined the potential of appreciative inquiry (AI) as a knowledge translation intervention in pain management nursing. The AI process focuses on an organization's strengths rather than weaknesses while looking for ways to improve practice. This makes it appealing to nurses because the traditional deficits approach to problem-solving can be perceived as demoralizing and punitive and could potentially result in resistance to change. AI is consistent with elements of the PARIHS framework; thus, this knowledge translation intervention could be grounded in theory which is integral to advancing knowledge translation in health care.

According to Kavanagh et al. (2008), the AI process could involve facilitated workshops with nurses on their units, and an affirmative topic could be introduced in the first phase, *Discovery*, by asking what is working well with respect to pain management practices. During the next phase, *Dream*, participants would select key factors that could enable them to practise evidence-based pain management. In the *Design* phase, nurses would articulate a clear vision for using pain management evidence on their unit. In the last phase, *Destiny*, they would develop an achievable action plan. Nurses do prefer dialogue with colleagues as a source of knowledge (Estabrooks et al. 2005), so this type of intervention during the workshops might be a realistic alternative to traditional ways of transferring knowledge about pain management practices.

10.7.8 Tailored Interventions

Tailored interventions are interventions planned following an investigation into the factors that explain current professional practice and any reasons for resisting new practice. One systematic review revealed that such interventions can change professional practice, though modestly (Baker et al. 2015). Another systematic review suggested that linking identified barriers to intervention component selection, while seeking input from staff about the acceptability of the intervention, may lead to changes in health-care providers' behaviour (Colquhoun et al. 2017).

Following a 3-year multiple site guideline implementation study by Higuchi et al. (2017), which included guidelines around pain management in addition to others, participants indicated that some of the process-related barriers to implementing practice guidelines were (a) increased workload demands, (b) competing organizational priorities, and (c) difficulty monitoring progress. Staff-related challenges included planning and scheduling meaningful education sessions, and organizational level barriers included infrastructure changes and administrative changes (Higuchi et al. 2017).

Ploeg et al. (2007) found that barriers to guideline implementation included negative staff attitudes and beliefs, limited integration of guideline recommendations into organizational structures and processes, time and resource constraints, and organizational and system level changes. If interventions can be tailored to target those barriers to change, adherence to guideline recommendations may be supported (Baker et al. 2015; Colquhoun et al. 2017). Facilitators of guideline implementation by 22 organizations, including pain assessment guidelines and six others, were (a) learning about the guidelines in small groups, (b) positive staff attitudes and beliefs related to change and the content of the guidelines, (c) leadership support which involved supporting the vision and providing staffing and other resources, (d) unit-based champions, (e) teamwork and collaboration, (f) financial support, and (e) interagency collaboration (Ploeg et al. 2007).

10.8   Sustaining Change

According to Roger's Diffusion of Innovations model, the decision to accept, adopt, and use an innovation such as a pain management guideline is influenced more by the nurse's perceptions of the guideline and less by how it is rated externally (Rogers 2003). The relative advantage of the guideline (i.e. whether it is perceived to be better than current practice), its compatibility with organizational values and capacities, and its complexity (i.e. perceptions of how difficult it is to use) all influence the rate of adoption (Rogers 2003).

Outlined in the National Health Service's sustainability model (Maher et al. 2007) are some factors that predict sustainability of practice change. In order of impact, they are (a) senior leadership engagement, (b) clinical leadership engagement, (c) staff involvement and training to sustain the process, (d) staff behaviours toward sustaining the change, (e) an organizational infrastructure for sustainability, (f) credibility of the evidence, (g) benefits beyond helping patients, (h) fit with the organization's strategic aims and culture, (i) adaptability of the improved process, and (j) effectiveness of the system to monitor progress.

In their study, Higuchi et al. (2017) noted that those implementing guidelines at eight study sites reported activities they had been using to support each of the ten factors outlined above. They generally included developing external partnerships, developing systems to monitor outcomes, chart audits, sharing progress, developing resources and educational sessions, and revising policies and systems.

Conclusion

Several barriers to pain management in older adults have been identified, and they may be addressed through implementation science. Successful knowledge translation relies on the use of a conceptual framework to guide the development, implementation, and sustainability of evidence-based pain management strategies. The Knowledge to Action and PARIHS frameworks lend themselves to this purpose.

Knowledge translation involves behaviour change, especially around nurses' decision-making. Some of the knowledge translation interventions applied to pain management are educational meetings, audit and feedback, reminders, opinion leaders and change champions, educational outreach, and appreciative inquiry. Tailoring interventions to address barriers can serve to support implementation of pain guideline recommendations. Barriers and facilitators (or determinants) of guideline uptake were outlined in this chapter along with factors impacting the sustainability of use of guidelines. Leadership involvement, credible evidence, staff buy-in and education, experiencing small successive "wins", and monitoring and feedback seem to be ingredients to successful implementation of pain management clinical practice guidelines.

References

American Geriatrics Society Panel on Persistent Pain in Older Persons. Management of persistent pain in older persons. J Am Geriatr Soc. 2002;50(6 Suppl):S205–24.

American Medical Directors Association. Pain management in the long term care setting. American Medical Directors Association (AMDA); 2012.

Australian Pain Society. Pain in residential aged care facilities-management strategies. 2005. https://www.apsoc.org.au/publications.

Baker R, Camosso-Stefinovic J, Gillies C, Shaw EJ, Cheater F, Flottorp S, et al. Tailored interventions to overcome identified barriers to change: effects on professional practice and health care outcomes. Cochrane Database Syst Rev. 2015. https://doi.org/10.1002/14651858.CD005470.pub3.

Brown D, McCormack B. Developing postoperative pain management: utilising the promoting action on research implementation in health services (PARIHS) framework. Worldviews Evid-Based Nurs. 2005;2(3):131–41. https://doi.org/10.1111/j.1741-6787.2005.00024.x.

Canadian Foundation for Healthcare Improvement. Glossary of knowledge exchange terms. 2017. http://www.cfhi-fcass.ca/PublicationsAndResources/ResourcesAndTools/GlossaryKnowledgeExchange.aspx.

Canadian Institutes of Health Research. Knowledge translation. 2016. http://www.cihr-irsc.gc.ca/e/29418.html.

Carlson C. Prior conditions influencing nurses' decisions to adopt evidence-based postoperative pain assessment practices. Pain Manag Nurs. 2010;11(4):245–58. https://doi.org/10.1016/j.pmn.2009.05.003.

Colquhoun HL, Squires JE, Kolehmainen N, Fraser C, Grimshaw JM. Methods for designing interventions to change healthcare professionals' behaviour: a systematic review. Implement Sci. 2017;12(1):30. https://doi.org/10.1186/s13012-017-0560-5.

Douglas C, Haydon D, Wollin J. Supporting staff to identify residents in pain: a controlled pretest-posttest study in residential aged care. Pain Manag Nurs. 2016;17(1):25–37. https://doi.org/10.1016/j.pmn.2015.08.001.

Drake G, Williams AC. Nursing education interventions for managing acute pain in hospital settings: A systematic review of clinical outcomes and teaching methods. Pain Manag Nurs. 2017;18(1):3–15. https://doi.org/10.1016/j.pmn.2016.11.001.

EPOC Taxonomy. Effective practice and organisation of care (EPOC). 2015. https://epoc.cochrane.org/epoc-taxonomy.

Ersek M, Neradilek MB, Herr K, Jablonski A, Polissar N, Du Pen A. Pain management algorithms for implementing best practices in nursing homes: results of a randomized controlled trial. J Am Med Dir Assoc. 2016;17(4):348–56. https://doi.org/10.1016/j.jamda.2016.01.001.

Estabrooks CA, Rutakumwa W, O'Leary KA, Profetto-McGrath J, Milner M, Levers MJ, et al. Sources of practice knowledge among nurses. Qual Health Res. 2005;15(4):460–76.

Etheridge F, Couturier Y, Denis J, Tremblay L, Tannenbaum C. Explaining the success or failure of quality improvement initiatives in long-term care organizations from a dynamic perspective. J Appl Gerontol. 2014;33(6):672–89. https://doi.org/10.1177/0733464813492582.

Feldman K, Berall A, Karuza J, Senderovich H, Perri G, Grossman D. Knowledge translation: an interprofessional approach to integrating a pain consult team within an acute care unit. J Interprof Care. 2016;30(6):816–8. https://doi.org/10.1080/13561820.2016.1195342.

Fleiszer A, Semenic S, Ritchie J, Richer M, Denis J. Nursing unit leaders' influence on the long-term sustainability of evidence-based practice improvements. J Nurs Manag. 2016;24(3):309–18. https://doi.org/10.1111/jonm.12320.

Foster R. Our incredible failure to incorporate evidence about pediatric pain management into clinical practice. J Spec Pediatr Nurs. 2013;18(3):171–2. https://doi.org/10.1111/jspn.12039.

Graham ID, Logan J, Harrison MB, Straus SE, Tetroe J, Caswell W, Robinson N. Lost in knowledge translation: time for a map? J Contin Educ Heal Prof. 2006;26(1):13–24. https://doi.org/10.1002/chp.47.

Greenhalgh T, Robert G, Macfarlane F, Bate P, Kyriakidou O. Diffusion of innovations in service organizations: systematic review and recommendations. Milbank Q. 2004;82(4):581–629. https://doi.org/10.1111/j.0887-378X.2004.00325.x.

Grimshaw J, Eccles M, Lavis J, Hill S, Squires J. Knowledge translation of research findings. Implement Sci. 2012;7:50. https://doi.org/10.1186/1748-5908-7-50.

Herr K, Coyne PJ, McCaffery M, Manworren R, Merkel S. Pain assessment in the patient unable to self-report: position statement with clinical practice recommendations. Pain Manag Nurs. 2011;12(4):230–50. https://doi.org/10.1016/j.pmn.2011.10.002.

Higuchi KS, Davies B, Ploeg J. Sustaining guideline implementation: a multisite perspective on activities, challenges and supports. J Clin Nurs. 2017;26:4413–24. https://doi.org/10.1111/jocn.13770.

Horgas AL, Yoon SL, Grall M. Pain management. In: Boltz M, Capezuti E, Fulmer T, Zwicker D, editors. Evidence-based geriatric nursing protocols for best practice. 4th ed. New York: Springer; 2012. p. 246–67.

Jeffs L, Indar A, Harvey B, McShane J, Bookey-Bassett S, Flintoft V, et al. Enabling role of manager in engaging clinicians and staff in quality improvement: being present and flexible. J Nurs Care Qual. 2016;31(4):367–72. https://doi.org/10.1097/NCQ.0000000000000196.

Kaasalainen S, Brazil K, Coker E, Ploeg J, Martin-Misener R, Donald F, et al. An action-based approach to improving pain management in long-term care. Can J Aging. 2010;29(4):503–17. https://doi.org/10.1017/S0714980810000528.

Kaasalainen S, Brazil K, Akhtar-Danesh N, Coker E, Ploeg J, Donald F, et al. The evaluation of an interdisciplinary pain protocol in long term care. J Am Med Dir Assoc. 2012;13(7):664.e1–8. https://doi.org/10.1016/j.jamda.2012.05.013.

Kaasalainen S, Ploeg J, Donald F, Coker E, Brazil K, Martin-Misener R, et al. Positioning clinical nurse specialists and nurse practitioners as change champions to implement a pain protocol in long-term care. Pain Manag Nurs. 2015;16(2):78–88. https://doi.org/10.1016/j.pmn.2014.04.002.

Kavanagh T, Stevens B, Seers K, Sidani S, Watt-Watson J. Examining appreciative inquiry as a knowledge translation intervention in pain management. Can J Nurs Res. 2008;40(2):40–56.

Maher L, Gustafson D, Evans A. Sustainability model and guide. NHS Institute for Innovation and Improvement; 2007.

Michie S, Johnston M, Abraham C, Lawton R, Parker D, Walker A. Making psychological theory useful for implementing evidence based practice: a consensus approach. Qual Saf Health Care. 2005;14(1):26–33. https://doi.org/10.1136/qshc.2004.011155.

Milat A, Li B. Narrative review of frameworks for translating research evidence into policy and practice. Public Health Res Pract. 2017;27:2711704. https://doi.org/10.17061/phrp2711704.

National Information Center on Health Services Research and Health Care Technology (NICHSR). Dissemination and implementation science. 2017. https://www.nlm.nih.gov/hsrinfo/implementation_science.html.

Nilsen P. Making sense of implementation theories, models and frameworks. Implement Sci. 2015;10(1):53. https://doi.org/10.1186/s13012-015-0242-0.

Ortiz MM, Carr E, Dikareva A. An integrative review of the literature on pain management barriers: implications for the Canadian clinical context. Can J Nurs Res. 2014;46(3):65–93.

Ploeg J, Davies B, Edwards N, Gifford W, Miller PE. Factors influencing best-practice guideline implementation: lessons learned from administrators, nursing staff, and project leaders. Worldviews Evid-Based Nurs. 2007;4(4):210–9. https://doi.org/10.1111/j.1741-6787.2007.00106.x.

Rogers EM. Diffusion of Innovations. 5th ed. New York: Free Press; 2003.

Rycroft-Malone J, Seers K, Chandler J, Hawkes CA, Crichton N, Allen C, et al. The role of evidence, context, and facilitation in an implementation trial: implications for the development of the PARIHS framework. Implement Sci. 2013;8(1):28. https://doi.org/10.1186/1748-5908-8-28.

Saunders H. Translating knowledge into best practice care bundles: a pragmatic strategy for EBP implementation via moving postprocedural pain management nursing guidelines into clinical practice. J Clin Nurs. 2015;24(13-14):2035–51. https://doi.org/10.1111/jocn.12812.

Savvas S, Toye C, Beattie E, Gibson S. Implementation of sustainable evidence-based practice for the assessment and management of pain in residential care facilities. Pain Manag Nurs. 2015;15:819–25. https://doi.org/10.1016/j.pmn.2013.09.002.

Schofield P, Sofaer-Bennett B, Hadjistavropoulos T, Zwakhalen S, Brown C, Westerling D, et al. A collaborative expert literature review of pain education, assessment and management. Aging Health. 2012;8(1):43–54.

Scott-Findlay S, Estabrooks C. Knowledge translation and pain management. In: Finley G, McGrath PJ, Chambers C, editors. Bringing pain relief to children: treatment approaches. Totowa: Humana; 2006. p. 199–227.

Song W, Eaton LH, Gordon DB, Hoyle C, Doorenbos AZ. Evaluation of evidence-based nursing pain management practice. Pain Manag Nurs. 2015;16(4):456–63. https://doi.org/10.1016/j.pmn.2014.09.001.

Stevens B. Challenges in knowledge translation: integrating evidence on pain in children into practice. Can J Nurs Res. 2009;41:109–14.

Swafford KL, Miller LL, Tsai PF, Herr KA, Ersek M. Improving the process of pain care in nursing homes: a literature synthesis. J Am Geriatr Soc. 2009;57(6):1080–7.

Twycross A. Educating nurses about pain management: the way forward. J Clin Nurs. 2002;11(6):705–14.

Yost J, Thompson D, Ganann R, Aloweni F, Newman K, McKibbon A, et al. Knowledge translation strategies for enhancing nurses' evidence-informed decision making: a scoping review. Worldviews Evid-Based Nurs. 2014;11(3):156–67. https://doi.org/10.1111/wvn.12043.

Zwakhalen SM, Hamers JP, Abu-Saad HH, Berger MP. Pain in elderly people with severe dementia: a systematic review of behavioural pain assessment tools. BMC Geriatr. 2006;6(1):3. https://doi.org/10.1186/1471-2318-6-3.